CONTENTS

INTRODUCTION

Growing up, I believed a great deal in magic. I always tried to stay up for Santa clause, and I knew my fairy Godmother was somewhere waiting for me to need her. But the source of magic that fascinated me most was my mother.

I remember watching her unpack groceries and take me out of the kitchen right before she started cooking. The next thing I know, she had completely transformed all those raw ingredients into a tantalizing meal that made everyone smile at the dinner table. She made all sorts of quick and tasty recipes that you can find in this cookbook, from my favorite fresh mixed fruit muffins to the delicious fruit crumble pie and zucchini pizza bites.

I would always beg her to teach me how she does it, but she would say, "when you're all grown up, darling." I longed for the day when I can magically turn ingredients into something that will brighten the hearts of my family.

Fast forward over 20 years. My mum gave me her book of recipes, I was old enough and ready to cook. Imagine my disappointment when every single meal I tried was a disaster. I got the right ingredients, followed the recipe closely, and yet my pizza crust was always so hard, and my garlic bread burnt. I decided after a while that maybe cooking just wasn't for me. Who would have thought I'd end up writing my very own cookbook?

I can never forget the day my mum came over for brunch, and I was making a simple lasagna toast. I was so embarrassed and couldn't understand why it came out with black edges until my mother told me the only problem was my oven.

How I Discovered the Black Decker Toaster Oven

I was so happy hearing I wasn't the problem. My cranky oven was to blame. I set out on a hunt for the best toaster oven for me. I read reviews, watched videos on YouTube, and was overwhelmed by all the information.

Finally, I called a couple of friends to find out their preferences. The one name that kept recurring was the Black Decker Toaster Oven. I knew I had to go on amazon and place an order swiftly. That was the one decision that transformed my cooking experience to date.

Every meal is as good as the appliance that you use in making it. It is safe to say, without the Black Decker toaster oven, I may have never written this cookbook. This purchase made it possible for me to explore my mum's recipes and create new ones that my kids can't get enough.

This cookbook comprises so many recipes that are sure to take you out of your comfort zone. The only way to ensure your effort is not in vain is by securing the best toaster oven for you.

Why This Cookbook Is the Best for You

Cooking is more than just throwing a bunch of stuff in a pot. You have to have the right ingredients in precise amounts subjected to a specific temperature for a given amount of time.

Cooking is chemistry, the way all the diverse elements combine to result in a bubbling or sizzling finish filling the air with a fresh aroma. Cooking is art, one meal can evoke different emotions from two people, and the same ingredients can mean various dishes depending on who is cooking.

Expect recipes that will require you to.

1. **Bake**

Most people hear the word "bake" and think of cake or bread! Get ready to be introduced to a whole new world of dishes you can bake that doesn't have flour as an ingredient. Yes, nothing can replace pastries, but baking isn't just about making cakes. So I put together diverse baking recipes.

The bulk of your work baking lies in the recipes which I have tailored to perfection for you. Make sure to check the number of servings per recipe. This way, you avoid lacking or wasting food, depending on the number of people you're expecting.Some of my favorite baking recipes included in this book are:

- Cheddar Breakfast Sausage Scones
- Orange-Glazed Whole Chicken
- Oven Baked Goulash
- Shrimp Fajitas with Avocado and Salsa
- Balsamic Prosciutto-Wrapped Asparagus
- Apple Pie with Caramel Sauce
- Rosemary Bread Loaf
- Italian Mozzarella Vegetable Pizza

Whether you love sweet or savory baking, the Black Decker toaster oven is just what you need.

2. **Broil**

Who needs a campfire to make s'mores when you have the Black Decker toaster oven? The best way to broil is to get your food at the right distance from the upper heat source. My last oven made it impossible for me to get the perfectly broiled chipotle tilapia because the rack position was just too close or too far away.

With the Black Decker toaster oven, I have a more compact space that puts my dish the right distance away from the upper heat element.

From a simple crispy sheet pan bacon to glazed pork tenderloin with veggies for dinner, the Black Decker toaster oven is my go-to for broiling. In this cookbook, you will see so many recipes that require broiling, like;

- Mozzarella Tomato Salsa Rounds
- Dijon-Rosemary Chicken Breasts
- Minted-Balsamic Lamb Chops
- Bourbon Sirloin Steak
- Lemon Torte with Cream Cheese Frosting
- Thin Crepes

There's no end to the possibilities of dishes you can create. After exploring all the recipes in this book, nothing stops you from thinking up recipes and trying them out. That was how I first came up with my famous broiled seafood platter, and now it's all my family wants to celebrate special occasions.

3. **Toast**

Nothing represents a quick, tasty, and effortless meal like a classic toast. But you can toast more than a few slices of bread with the Black Decker toaster oven. My former toaster didn't inspire me to explore this section due to its faulty temperature regulation.

Most of the toast recipes in this cookbook still save me, especially on days when I have no time to cook whole meals for my kids to take to school. I just whip up a healthy and filling recipe like the Toasted Ham and apple sandwich that keeps my kids satisfied until they're back home.

Other recipes that will go perfectly with your Black Decker toaster oven are:

- Sausage French Toast Casserole with Maple
- Peppery Smoked Turkey and Walnut Sandwich
- Portable Cheesy Bacon Omelet
- Lamb Leg with Herb Yogurt Sauce

Also, expect to see various toast ideas that are also perfect for vegans. Some toast recipes include;

- Mincemeat and Cranberry Stuffed Apple
- Vegetarian Portobello Burgers

The recipes I put together in this cookbook are straightforward and easy to make. With the Black Decker toaster oven, you'll be whipping up incredible meals like it's nothing. It doesn't matter if you are new to the kitchen scene or have been cooking for years.

4. **Warm**

Nothing wrong with leaving a little leftover for the next day. They often come in handy for me on weekends when I want to sleep in and not have to prepare breakfast for my family. Also, my husband loves having his early morning plate of leftover apple pie with fruit juice.

Why throw out leftovers when you can warm to taste almost as good as when you first had them? This remarkable reheating capacity is one that the Black Decker toaster oven is renowned for. My chicken BBQ pizza tastes juicy and crisp days after I prepared it.

After my first try using this oven, I totally abandoned my microwave. All it did was make my meals either too dry or soggy when reheating. Think of the Black Decker toaster oven as a "Smart" oven that makes amazing and crunchy toasts as well.

Why Should You Choose the Black Decker Toaster Oven?

There are a bunch of toaster ovens on the market that promise you this, that, and the other. Why the Black Decker Toaster oven should be your top pick is quite simple. Here are 6 essential reasons;

1. Won't Cost You a Fortune

I was reluctant about getting a toaster oven at first because I thought it would cost a lot. My husband and I had a lot of bills to pay, and I wasn't about to break the bank to buy a kitchen appliance. I was so delighted to discover how affordable the Black Decker toaster oven was. Frankly, I thought I'd have to start saving to make a purchase, but I ended up placing an order that same day.

Who doesn't love a good deal? Especially one that does not come at the expense of quality and durability. I have been using my Black Decker toaster oven for years now, and I've never had to take it for any form of repairs. My former toaster oven was either electrocuting someone or needing an adaptor change.

If you are looking for a cost-effective companion to create all the meals I have lined up for you? Then you should go for the Black Decker toaster oven. It will save you a few bucks and still have you preparing great dishes.

2. Easy to Use

The side menu on the Black Decker toaster has all its functions clearly stated. The menu it came with was straightforward and easy to understand, that I didn't hesitate to make garlic bread the same day it arrived. Why have a device you can't use efficiently? Depending on your recipe, you will need to regulate the temperature, set cooking mode, and also time your food. My former toaster oven felt like a crossword puzzle (and not the fun type) that had me dreading my kitchen.

3. Temperature Regulation and Timer

I was astonished to see that the Black Decker toaster oven reaches up to 450 degrees with accurate temperature regulation. That way, I determine how much heat each dish needs for a set amount of time.

Cooking no longer requires my 100% attention. I can leave my sliced baguette in the oven and get a little work done because I know there's no chance of it getting burnt. Even my husband noticed I stopped running to the kitchen since I got the Black Decker toaster oven. Everyone forgets while cooking once in a while. You don't deserve to skip dinner for that.

4. Easy to Move About

This advantage is one that all mothers will cherish. As long as you have healthy kids in your house, expect them to press things. My son went through a phase that my husband and I named the "Button magnet" phase. Junior went about pushing anything that remotely resembled a button.

We had to use the lock on the kitchen door, but they can't stay shut forever. I wasn't too bothered because I had the option of placing my Black Decker toaster oven in a cabinet that's high up. I could quickly bring it down whenever I wanted to use it and return after use.

5. Easy to Clean

Your health starts in your kitchen. Not only is a clean kitchen healthy, it automatically makes your cooking experience more enjoyable. Cleaning up Bread crumbs, melted cheese, bits of chicken, and drips of a marinade from the Black Decker toaster oven has been extremely easy for me. The removable crumb tray and flexible door make it easy to maneuver to all those corners that tend to store up dirt over time.

6. Big Enough for Your Family

You may be concerned about space, I was too. Imagine my pleasure when I found out this versatile toaster oven came in different sizes. So if like me, you cook for a big family, you should opt for the Extra-wide convection toaster oven as opposed to the regular-sized toaster oven.

Wrap Up

I specially designed all the recipes in this book to make your recreation of delicious dishes effortless. Your journey through these meals will only be as enjoyable as the quality of your kitchen. No need to panic, you don't have to spend a lot of money buying all new kitchen appliances, but there's nothing as good as a worthy investment.

All you'll be needed is the Black Decker toaster oven to make virtually all the recipes in this book. You can do much more with this oven than toast a couple of bread slices. Gone are the days when you focus on just the 'toast' part as this equipment is getting better and smarter.

CHAPTER 1 BREAKFAST

Maple Oats and Nuts

Prep time: 15 minutes | Cook time: 35 minutes | Makes 7 to 8 cups

3 cups old-fashioned rolled oats (use gluten-free if necessary)
¾ cup shredded sweetened coconut
¾ cup raw cashews
¾ cup chopped raw walnuts
½ cup pumpkin seeds
¼ cup sesame seeds (optional)
¼ cup dark brown sugar
½ cup maple syrup
¼ cup oil (coconut, grapeseed, safflower, or other neutral-flavored oil with a high smoke point)
1 teaspoon ground cinnamon
1 teaspoon vanilla extract
¾ teaspoon kosher salt
1 cup raisins

1. Select Convection Bake and preheat the oven to 275ºF (135ºC).
2. Position two racks at even intervals from the oven's top and bottom, and each other.
3. In a large bowl, stir together the oats, coconut, cashews, walnuts, pumpkin seeds, sesame seeds (if using), and brown sugar.
4. In a small bowl, stir together the maple syrup, oil, cinnamon, vanilla, and salt. Add the wet maple syrup mixture to the oat-nut mixture and stir to mix well. Divide the nut mixture between two rimmed baking sheets and spread it in an even layer. Bake both sheets together for 35 to 40 minutes, stirring once or twice, until the oats and nuts are golden brown.
5. Transfer the hot mixture to a large bowl and immediately stir in the raisins. Cool to room temperature before serving or storing.

Brown Sugar Pastries with Cinnamon

Prep time: 15 minutes | Cook time: 20 minutes | Makes 4 pastries

For the Filling:
¼ cup light brown sugar
2 teaspoons ground cinnamon
1 tablespoon all-purpose flour
For the Dough:
2½ cups all-purpose flour, plus more for rolling the dough
2 teaspoons sugar
1 teaspoon table salt
1 cup cold, unsalted butter, cut into small pieces
4 to 6 tablespoons ice-cold water
1 large egg
1 tablespoon water
For the Topping:
¾ cup confectioners' sugar
½ teaspoon ground cinnamon
1 teaspoon vanilla extract
4 teaspoons milk

Make the Filling

1. In a small bowl, stir together the brown sugar, cinnamon, and flour. Set aside.

Make the Dough

2. In a large bowl, stand mixer, or food processor, combine the flour, sugar, and salt. Stir or pulse to mix.
3. Add the butter. Using a pastry cutter, two knives, or a mixing blade attachment on your mixer, cut it into the flour until the mixture begins to come together in crumbs.
4. Slowly add the water, 1 tablespoon at a time, while stirring or with the mixer or food processor running, until the dough balls up and begins to pull away from the sides of the bowl. Remove the dough and form it into 2 equal-size disks. Wrap each in plastic wrap and refrigerate for at least 30 minutes.
5. Select Convection Bake and preheat the oven to 350ºF (180ºC).
6. Line a baking sheet with parchment paper.
7. Unwrap one of the dough disks and, on a floured board and using a rolling pin, roll it into a roughly 9-by-12-inch rectangle, an even ⅛ inch thick. Cut the rectangle into 4 (4½-by-3-inch) rectangles

and place them on the prepared sheet. Refrigerate the rectangles while you roll and cut the remaining dough disk in the same manner.

8. Once you have 8 (3-by-4-inch) rectangles, in a small bowl, whisk the egg and water. Brush a bit of the egg wash over the rectangles.

9. Place 1 heaping tablespoon of filling on each of 4 egg-washed rectangles and spread it to cover the pastry to within about ¼ inch of the edge, leaving a border for sealing two pieces of dough together.

10. Top each filled rectangle with 1 egg-washed rectangle, egg wash–side down. Use the tines of a fork to press and seal the edges together all the way around. Use the tip of a sharp knife to poke several holes in the pastry to let steam escape as they bake.

11. Bake for 16 to 20 minutes, until the tops are golden brown. Remove from the oven and let the pastries cool for about 10 minutes on the pan before transferring them to a wire rack to cool completely.

Make the Topping

12. In a small bowl, stir together the confectioners' sugar, cinnamon, vanilla, and milk. Once the pastries are nearly or completely cool, drizzle the topping mixture decoratively over the tops. Serve slightly warm or at room temperature.

Chocolate Coffee Cake with Pecan

Prep time: 15 minutes | Cook time: 35 minutes | Serves 12

For the Topping:

¾ cup all-purpose flour
¾ cup dark brown sugar
½ teaspoon table salt
¾ cup chopped pecans
6 tablespoons unsalted butter, cubed

For the Chocolate Swirl:

½ cup sugar
1 tablespoon unsweetened cocoa powder

For the Cake

1 cup unsalted butter, at room temperature, plus more for preparing the pan
3½ cups all-purpose flour
1½ teaspoons baking soda
1 teaspoon baking powder
½ teaspoon table salt
2 cups sugar
4 large eggs
16 ounces (454 g) sour cream
1½ teaspoons vanilla extract

Make the Topping

1. In a food processor, combine the flour, brown sugar, salt, and pecans and pulse until finely chopped.

2. Add the butter and pulse until the mixture resembles coarse crumbs.

Make the Chocolate Swirl

3. In a small bowl, stir together the sugar and cocoa powder.

Make the Cake

4. Select Convection Bake and preheat the oven to 325ºF (163ºC).

5. Butter a 9-by-13-inch baking pan.

6. In a medium bowl, whisk the flour, baking soda, baking powder, and salt.

7. In a large bowl, using an electric mixer, beat the butter on medium speed until creamy and smooth.

8. Add the sugar and beat until the mixture is fluffy and light yellow.

9. Add the eggs, one a time, beating after each addition just until incorporated.

10. Add the sour cream and vanilla and beat to combine.

11. Add the flour mixture in three batches, beating just to combine after each addition. Transfer about one-third of the cake batter to the prepared pan and spread it into an even layer. Sprinkle half the chocolate swirl mixture over the batter. Top with half the remaining batter and all of the remaining chocolate swirl mixture. Add all the remaining cake batter to the pan and gently spread it evenly over the top.

12. Sprinkle the topping mixture evenly over the entire top of the cake.

13. Bake for 35 to 45 minutes, until the topping is golden brown and a toothpick inserted into the center of the cake comes out clean.

14. Set the baking pan on a wire rack and let the cake cool completely before serving.

Cheddar Breakfast Sausage Scones

Prep time: 10 minutes | Cook time: 15 minutes | Serves 6

1½ cups all-purpose flour
2 teaspoons baking powder
½ teaspoon kosher salt
3 tablespoons unsalted butter, very cold
1 cup coarsely grated sharp Cheddar cheese
2 or 3 scallions, finely chopped
8 ounces (227 g) breakfast sausage, cooked and coarsely chopped
1 large egg, beaten, divided
½ cup heavy (whipping) cream

1. Select Convection Bake and preheat the oven to 425ºF (220ºC). Line a sheet pan with a silicone baking mat.
2. In a large bowl, whisk together the flour, baking powder, and salt. Using the large holes of a cheese grater, grate the butter into the flour mixture and stir to combine. Mix in the cheese, scallions, and sausage.
3. Pour 1 tablespoon of the beaten egg into a small bowl and set aside. Whisk the cream into the remaining egg. Add the egg mixture to the flour and butter mixture. The dough should hold together but be shaggy rather than moist.
4. Transfer the dough to a lightly floured work surface. Gather it together into a rectangle. Fold the dough into thirds and press together. Repeat.
5. Form the dough into a smooth 6-inch disk. Cut the disk into 6 wedges, and carefully transfer them to the prepared pan.
6. Brush the scones with the reserved egg.
7. Bake for 15 to 18 minutes, until golden brown, rotating halfway through if they're browning unevenly. Cool on the pan for about 10 minutes. Serve warm or at room temperature.

Dutch Baby with Mixed Berries Topping

Prep time: 10 minutes | Cook time: 20 minutes | Serves 4

3 tablespoons unsalted butter, at room temperature
¾ cup whole milk
3 large eggs
½ cup all-purpose flour
¼ cup sugar, plus 2 tablespoons
½ teaspoon vanilla extract
¼ teaspoon kosher salt
1 (10- to 12-ounce / 283- to 340-g) package frozen mixed berries, thawed
1 tablespoon freshly squeezed lemon juice

1. Select Bake and preheat the oven to 425ºF (220ºC). Put the butter in a 10-inch cast-iron skillet and place it in the oven while the oven heats.
2. Meanwhile, make the batter. In a blender (or in a large bowl with a hand mixer), combine the milk, eggs, flour, the 2 tablespoons of sugar, vanilla, and salt and blend until smooth.
3. When the oven is at temperature and the butter in the skillet has stopped foaming, remove the skillet from the oven and pour in the batter.
4. Turn the oven to Convection Bake and reduce the temperature to 400ºF (205ºC). Bake for 20 minutes without opening the oven. The pancake should be puffed and golden brown, with darker brown edges. Bake for another 5 minutes if necessary.
5. Meanwhile, pour the berries and their juices into a small bowl. Add the remaining ¼ cup of sugar and the lemon juice, and stir to dissolve the sugar.
6. When the pancake is done, slice into wedges and serve with a scoop of berries on top.

Swiss Ham Mustard Pastries

Prep time: 10 minutes | Cook time: 20 minutes | Serves 4

¾ cup diced ham
½ cup shredded Gruyère or other Swiss-style cheese
2 tablespoons cream cheese, softened
1 tablespoon Dijon mustard
1 sheet frozen puff pastry, thawed
1 large egg, beaten
2 tablespoons finely grated Parmesan cheese

1. Select Convection Bake and preheat the oven to 350ºF (180ºC). Line a sheet pan with a silicone baking mat.
2. In a medium bowl, stir together the ham, shredded cheese, cream cheese, and mustard.

3. Lightly flour a cutting board. Unfold the puff pastry sheet onto the board. Using a rolling pin, gently roll the dough to smooth out the folds, sealing any tears. Cut the dough into four squares.

4. Scoop a quarter of the ham mixture into the center of each puff pastry square and spread it evenly in a triangle shape over half the pastry, leaving a ½-inch border around the edges. Fold the pastry diagonally over the filling to form triangles. With a fork, crimp the edges to seal them. Place the pastries on the prepared pan, spacing them evenly.

5. Cut two or three small slits into the top of each turnover. Brush with the egg and sprinkle the Parmesan on top.

6. Bake for 10 to 12 minutes, then remove from the oven. Check the pastries; if they are browning unevenly, rotate the pan. Return the pan to the oven and continue baking for another 10 minutes, or until the turnovers are golden brown.

7. Let cool for about 10 minutes before serving (the filling will be very hot).

Sausage French Toast Casserole with Maple

Prep time: 5 minutes | Cook time: 45 minutes | Serves 4

6 fresh breakfast sausage links
4 large eggs
1½ cups whole milk
½ teaspoon kosher salt
5 tablespoons pure maple syrup, divided
5 or 6 thick slices of stale bread, cut into 1-inch cubes

1. Select Bake and preheat the oven to 375ºF (190ºC).

2. Put the sausage links in oven and bake for about 15 minutes, until lightly browned. They may not be cooked all the way through, but they will cook again. You just want to render some of their fat.

3. Meanwhile, in a medium bowl, whisk the eggs until completely mixed. Add the milk, salt, and 1 tablespoon of maple syrup and whisk to combine. Add the bread cubes and gently stir to coat with the egg mixture. Let sit for 2 to 3 minutes to let the bread absorb some of the custard, then gently stir again.

4. After the sausages have browned, remove the oven. Turn the oven to Convection Bake and reduce the temperature to 350ºF (180ºC). Transfer the sausages to a plate. If there is more than a thin coat of fat on the bottom of the pot, pour out the excess.

5. Pour the bread mixture into the oven, then top with the sausage links.

6. Bake for 30 minutes, or until the sausages are browned and a knife inserted into the center of the casserole comes out clean.

7. Serve with the remaining 4 tablespoons of maple syrup.

Mozzarella Tomato Salsa Rounds

Prep time: 5 minutes | Cook time: 6 minutes | Makes 12 slices

1 French baguette, cut to make 12
1-inch slices (rounds)
¼ cup olive oil
1 cup tomato salsa
½ cup shredded low-fat Mozzarella
2 tablespoons finely chopped fresh cilantro

1. Brush both sides of each round with olive oil.

2. Spread one side of each slice with salsa and sprinkle each with Mozzarella. Place the rounds in an oiled or nonstick 8½ × 8½ × 2-inch square baking (cake) pan.

3. Broil for 6 minutes, or until the cheese is melted and the rounds are lightly browned. Garnish with the chopped cilantro and serve.

Vegetarian Portobello Burgers

Prep time: 10 minutes | Cook time: 12 minutes | Serves 4

4 multigrain hamburger buns Dijon mustard
4 large portobello mushroom caps, stemmed and brushed clean
2 tablespoons olive oil
Garlic powder
Salt and butcher's pepper, to taste
4 thin onion slices
4 tomato slices

1. Toast the split hamburger buns and spread each slice with mustard. Set aside.

2. Brush both sides of the mushroom caps with olive oil and sprinkle with garlic powder and salt and pepper to taste.

3. Broil the caps on a broiling rack with a pan underneath, ribbed side up, for 6 minutes. Turn the mushrooms carefully with tongs and broil again for 6 minutes, or until lightly browned. Place the mushroom caps on the bottom buns and layer each with an onion and tomato slice. Top with the remaining bun halves and serve.

Peppery Smoked Turkey and Walnut Sandwich

Prep time: 10 minutes | Cook time: 5 minutes | Serves 2

Stone-ground mustard
2 tablespoons canned diced pimientos
2 tablespoons finely chopped scallions
2 tablespoons finely chopped walnuts
2 tablespoons chopped raisins
½ teaspoon dill
2 tablespoons reduced-fat mayonnaise
Salt and butcher's pepper, to taste
4 slices rye bread
1 (2½-ounce / 71-g) package smoked turkey breast slices

1. Combine the mixture ingredients and spread in equal portions on all bread slices. Layer 2 bread slices with equal portions of smoked turkey breast. Top with the other bread slices to make sandwiches.

2. Toast twice on a broiling rack with a pan underneath.

Almond, Coconut, and Apple Granola

Prep time: 10 minutes | Cook time: 12 minutes | Serves 6

3 cups gluten-free old-fashioned rolled oats
1 cup slivered almonds
1 cup unsweetened coconut chips
½ cup honey or pure maple syrup
$^{1}/_{3}$ cup packed light brown sugar
¼ cup vegetable oil
1 teaspoon ground cinnamon
¼ teaspoon kosher salt
2 cups chopped dried apples

1. Select Convection Bake and preheat the oven to 325ºF (163ºC).

2. In a large bowl, combine the oats, almonds, coconut, honey, brown sugar, oil, cinnamon, and salt and mix well. Spread the mixture in an even layer on a sheet pan.

3. Bake for 6 minutes. Remove the pan and stir the granola. Return to the oven and continue baking until the nuts and oats are golden brown and crisp, another 6 to 8 minutes.

4. Let cool, then stir in the apples.

Orange Cranberry Muffins

Prep time: 15 minutes | Cook time: 25 minutes | Serves 12

Nonstick cooking spray
2¼ cups all-purpose flour
¾ cup sugar
2 teaspoons baking powder
Finely grated zest and juice of 1 orange
½ teaspoon kosher salt
¼ teaspoon baking soda
10 tablespoons unsalted butter, at room temperature, cut into ½-inch pieces
¼ cup whole milk
2 large eggs
1 teaspoon vanilla extract
1 cup dried cranberries

1. Select Convection Bake and preheat the oven to 350ºF (180ºC). Coat a 12-cup muffin tin with cooking spray.

2. Combine the flour, sugar, baking powder, orange zest, salt, baking soda, and butter in the bowl of a stand mixer with a paddle attachment (or use a hand mixer). Mix on low speed for about 2 minutes, until the butter has broken into very small clumps. The mixture will look powdery but hold together when pinched.

3. Add the milk, orange juice, eggs, and vanilla. Mix on low just until combined and very thick.

4. Stir in the cranberries.

5. Divide the batter evenly among the prepared muffin cups. Bake until the muffins are puffed, golden brown, and firm to the touch, about 25

minutes, rotating the tin after 15 minutes if cooking unevenly.

Parmesan Ham and Egg Cups

Prep time: 5 minutes | Cook time: 12 minutes | Serves 6

Nonstick cooking spray
6 thin slices ham
6 large eggs
Kosher salt, to taste
Freshly ground black pepper, to taste
2 tablespoons finely grated Parmesan cheese

1. Select Bake and preheat the oven to 375ºF (190ºC).
2. Spray the cups of a 6-cup muffin tin with cooking spray. Press a slice of ham into each cup, smoothing out the sides as much as possible. The ham should extend over the top of the cup by ¼ to ½ inch. Crack an egg into each cup and season with salt and pepper. Top each yolk with 1 teaspoon of the cheese.
3. Bake for 5 minutes, then slide out the rack and check the eggs. They should just be starting to firm up and turn opaque. Rotate the muffin tin if the eggs are cooking unevenly.
4. Cook for another 5 minutes and check again; if the egg whites are cooked through, remove the tin from the oven. The total cook time is about 12 minutes for fully cooked whites and runny yolks; if you prefer the yolks more done, cook for an additional minute or two.
5. When the eggs are cooked as desired, remove the muffin tin and let cool for a couple of minutes. Run a thin knife around the ham and use a spoon to remove the cups.

Mozzarella Herby Smoked Salmon Frittata

Prep time: 10 minutes | Cook time: 13 minutes | Serves 4

2 tablespoons unsalted butter
¼ cup chopped onion
8 large eggs
½ teaspoon kosher salt
¼ cup whole milk
2 tablespoons chopped fresh dill
2 tablespoons chopped fresh chives
1 tablespoon chopped fresh parsley
3 ounces (85 g) smoked salmon, flaked or chopped
½ cup grated Mozzarella cheese
¼ teaspoon freshly ground black pepper

1. Select Bake and preheat the oven to 375ºF (190ºC).
2. In an oven-safe nonstick or cast-iron skillet, heat the butter over medium-high heat until foaming. Add the onion and cook, stirring occasionally, for about 5 minutes, or until soft.
3. While the onion cooks, whisk the eggs with the salt in a medium bowl. Let sit for a minute or two, then add the milk and whisk again until the eggs are thoroughly mixed with no streaks of white remaining, but not foamy. Stir in the dill, chives, and parsley.
4. Distribute the salmon evenly over the bottom of the skillet with the onion. Pour the egg mixture into the pan. Let the eggs cook, undisturbed, for 5 to 7 minutes, until the edges are set. The center will still be quite liquid. If the frittata begins to form large bubbles on the bottom, use a silicone spatula to break them up.
5. Run a silicone spatula around the edges of the frittata. Transfer the skillet to the oven and bake for about 2 minutes, until the center is just set. Remove the skillet from the oven and sprinkle the cheese over the top. Return the pan to the oven and bake for another 1 to 2 minutes, until the cheese is melted and very slightly browned. Sprinkle the pepper over the frittata.
6. Let the frittata rest for 1 to 2 minutes. To serve, either divide the frittata into four wedges in the skillet, or run the spatula around the edges again and slide the whole frittata out onto a plate before cutting it into wedges. Serve warm or at room temperature.

Baked Fries with Bacon and Eggs

Prep time: 10 minutes | Cook time: 23 minutes | Serves 4

2 medium Yukon gold potatoes, peeled and cut into ¼-inch cubes (about 3 cups)
1 medium onion, chopped

$^{1}/_{3}$ cup diced red or green bell pepper
1 tablespoon vegetable oil
½ teaspoon kosher salt, divided
¼ teaspoon freshly ground black pepper, divided
12 ounces (340 g) thick-sliced bacon, cut into ¼-inch pieces
4 large eggs

1. Select Bake and preheat the oven to 375ºF (190ºC).
2. Put the potatoes, onion, and bell pepper on a sheet pan. Drizzle with the oil, ¼ teaspoon of salt, and ⅛ teaspoon of pepper and toss to coat. Spread the vegetables out in a single layer as much as possible. Scatter the bacon pieces evenly over the top.
3. Bake for 10 minutes, then remove the pan from the oven and stir the potato mixture. Return to the oven and bake for another 10 minutes, or until the potatoes are tender inside and beginning to crisp on the outside, and the bacon is becoming crisp.
4. Remove the pan from the oven. Using a large spoon, create four circular openings in the potato mixture. Gently crack an egg into each opening; season the eggs with the remaining ¼ teaspoon of salt and ⅛ teaspoon of pepper. Return the pan to the oven and bake for 3 minutes for very runny yolks or up to 8 minutes for firm yolks.
5. Use a spatula to transfer the eggs from the pan to four separate plates, then scoop out the home fries to serve on the side.

Sweet Banana Bread

Prep time: 10 minutes | Cook time: 40 minutes | Serves 6

2 ripe bananas
1 egg
½ cup skim milk
2 tablespoons honey
1 tablespoon vegetable oil
1 cup unbleached flour
¾ cup chopped trail mix
1 teaspoon baking powder
Salt, to taste

1. Preheat the toaster oven to 400ºF (205ºC).
2. Process the bananas, egg, milk, honey, and oil in a blender or food processor until smooth and transfer to a mixing bowl.
3. Add the flour and trail mix, stirring to mix well. Add the baking powder and stir just enough to blend it into the batter. Add Salt, to taste. Pour the mixture into an oiled or nonstick 4½ × 8½ × 2¼-inch loaf pan.
4. Bake for 40 minutes, or until a toothpick inserted in the center comes out clean.

Half-and-Half Cinnamon Rolls

Prep time: 10 minutes | Cook time: 15 minutes | Makes 12 rolls and ½ cup icing

Cinnamon Mixture:

3 tablespoons dark brown sugar
3 tablespoons chopped pecans
2 tablespoons margarine
1 teaspoon ground cinnamon
Salt, to taste

Icing:

1 cup confectioners' sugar, sifted
1 tablespoon fat-free half-and-half
½ teaspoon vanilla extract
Salt, to taste

1. Preheat the toaster oven to 400ºF (205ºC).
2. Make the buttermilk biscuit dough.
3. Roll out or pat the dough to ½ inch thick. In a small bowl, combine the cinnamon mixture ingredients. Spread the dough evenly with the cinnamon mixture and roll up like a jelly roll. With a sharp knife, cut the roll into 1-inch slices. Place on an oiled or nonstick 6½ × 10-inch baking sheet.
4. Bake for 15 minutes, or until lightly browned. Let cool before frosting.
5. Combine the icing ingredients in a small bowl, adding more half-and-half or confectioners' sugar until the consistency is like thick cream. Drizzle over the tops of the cinnamon rolls and serve.

Low-Fat Buttermilk Biscuits

Prep time: 10 minutes | Cook time: 15 minutes | Makes 12 biscuits

2 cups unbleached flour
1 tablespoon baking powder
½ teaspoon baking soda
Salt, to taste
3 tablespoons margarine, at room temperature
1 cup low-fat buttermilk

Vegetable oil

1. Preheat the toaster oven to 400ºF (205ºC).
2. Combine the flour, baking powder, baking soda, and Salt, to taste in a medium bowl.
3. Cut in the margarine with 2 knives or a pastry blender until the mixture is crumbly.
4. Stir in the buttermilk, adding just enough so the dough will stay together when pinched.
5. Knead the dough on a floured surface for one minute, then pat or roll out the dough to ¾ inch thick. Cut out biscuit rounds with a 2½-inch biscuit cutter. Place the rounds on an oiled or nonstick 6½ × 10-inch baking sheet.
6. Bake for 15 minutes, or until golden brown.

Breakfast Raisins Bars

Prep time: 15 minutes | Cook time: 35 minutes | Makes 6 bars

1 cup unsweetened applesauce
1 carrot, peeled and grated
½ cup raisins
1 egg
1 tablespoon vegetable oil
2 tablespoons molasses
2 tablespoons brown sugar
¼ cup chopped walnuts
2 cups rolled oats
2 tablespoons sesame seeds
1 teaspoon ground cinnamon
¼ teaspoon grated nutmeg
¼ teaspoon ground ginger
Salt, to taste

1. Preheat the toaster oven to 375ºF (190ºC).
2. Combine all the ingredients in a bowl, stirring well to blend. Press the mixture into an oiled or nonstick 8½ × 8½ × 2inch square baking (cake) pan.
3. Bake for 35 minutes, or until golden brown. Cool and cut into squares.

Coffee Cake with Pecan

Prep time: 10 minutes | Cook time: 40 minutes | Serves 6

For the Cake:
2 cups unbleached flour
2 teaspoons baking powder
2 tablespoons vegetable oil
1 egg
1¼ cups skim milk

For the Topping:
½ cup brown sugar
1 tablespoon margarine, at room temperature
1 teaspoon ground cinnamon
¼ teaspoon grated nutmeg
¼ cup chopped pecans
Salt, to taste

1. Preheat the toaster oven to 375ºF (190ºC).
2. Combine the ingredients for the cake in a medium bowl and mix thoroughly. Pour the batter into an oiled or 8½ × 8½ × 2inch square baking (cake) pan and set aside.
3. Combine the topping ingredients in a small bowl, mashing the margarine into the dry ingredients with a fork until the mixture is crumbly. Sprinkle evenly on top of the batter.
4. Bake for 40 minutes, or until a toothpick inserted in the center comes out clean. Cool and cut into squares.

Portable Cheesy Bacon Omelet

Prep time: 5 minutes | Cook time: 4 minutes | Serves 1

2 slices multigrain bread
2 eggs
1 tablespoon plain nonfat yogurt
Salt and freshly ground black pepper, to taste
2 strips turkey bacon
2 tablespoons shredded low-moisture, part-skim Mozzarella cheese

1. Toast the bread slices and set aside.
2. Whisk together the eggs and yogurt in a small bowl and season with salt and pepper to taste.
3. Layer bacon strips in a small 4 × 8 × 2¼-inch loaf pan. Pour the egg mixture on top and sprinkle with the cheese.
4. Toast once, or until the egg is done to your preference. Cut the omelet into toast-size squares and place between the 2 slices of toast to make a sandwich.

Whole Wheat Mozzarella Pita

Prep time: 5 minutes | Cook time: 3 minutes | Serves 2

1 (5-inch) whole wheat pita loaf
1 teaspoon olive oil
1 egg, well beaten
2 tablespoons shredded low-fat Mozzarella cheese
Garlic powder
Salt and freshly ground black pepper

1. Cut a circle out of the top layer of one pita bread loaf and remove the disk-shaped layer, leaving the bottom intact. Brush the pita loaf with the olive oil. Carefully pour the beaten egg into the cavity. Sprinkle with cheese and season with garlic powder and salt and pepper to taste.
2. Toast once on the oven rack, or until the egg is cooked thoroughly and the cheese is lightly browned.

Homemade Gypsy Lights

Prep time: 5 minutes | Cook time: 4 minutes | Serves 1

1 slice multigrain bread
1 teaspoon vegetable oil
1 egg
Salt and freshly ground black pepper, to taste

1. Brush both sides of bread with the oil and place in a 6½ × 6½ × 2-inch square (cake) pan. Cut or tear a circle of bread out of the center (the circle should be about 1½ inches across). Place the circle in the pan also.
2. Pour the egg into the cavity in the center of the bread. Season to taste with salt and pepper.
3. Toast twice, or until the egg is done to your preference.

Perfect Sunny-Side up Eggs

Prep time: 5 minutes | Cook time: 3 minutes | Serves 2

2 large eggs
Salt and freshly ground black pepper, to taste

1. Crack the eggs into an oiled or nonstick small 4 × 8 × 2¼-inch loaf pan. Sprinkle with salt and pepper to taste.
2. Toast once, or until the eggs are done to your preference.

Creamy Parmesan Eggs

Prep time: 5 minutes | Cook time: 10 minutes | Serves 4

4 large eggs, each cracked into a small 1-cup baking dish
4 tablespoons grated Parmesan cheese
4 tablespoons fat-free half-and-half
Salt and freshly ground black pepper, to taste

1. Preheat the toaster oven to 400ºF (205ºC).
2. Top each egg with 1 tablespoon Parmesan cheese and 1 tablespoon half-and-half. Season to taste with salt and pepper and add any preferred additions.
3. Bake for 10 minutes, or to your preference, testing the eggs by touching the surface with a spoon for the desired firmness after 5 minutes.

CHAPTER 2 POULTRY

Feta Spinach Stuffed Chicken Breast

Prep time: 15 minutes | Cook time: 35 minutes | Serves 4

Nonstick cooking spray, for preparing the pan and rack

For the Filling:

4 ounces (113 g) cream cheese, at room temperature
2 ounces (57 g) crumbled Feta cheese
1 cup chopped fresh baby spinach
2 scallions, white and green parts, thinly sliced
3 garlic cloves, minced
½ teaspoon red pepper flakes
½ teaspoon kosher salt
¼ teaspoon freshly ground black pepper

For the Chicken Breasts:

4 (6-ounce / 170-g) boneless skinless chicken breasts
2 large eggs, lightly beaten
1½ cups panko bread crumbs
½ cup freshly grated Parmesan cheese
½ teaspoon Italian seasoning
¼ teaspoon kosher salt
¼ teaspoon freshly ground black pepper

1. Select Convection Bake and preheat the oven to 350ºF (180ºC).
2. Place a wire rack on top of a baking sheet and spray both with cooking spray.

Make the Filling

3. In a medium bowl, stir together the cream cheese, Feta, spinach, scallions, garlic, red pepper flakes, salt, and pepper. Set aside.

Make the Chicken Breasts

4. Make a horizontal cut most of the way through each chicken breast to make a pocket for the filling. Cover the chicken with plastic wrap or parchment paper and pound out each piece so it is a nearly even ½ inch thick.
5. Spoon one-fourth of the filling into the pocket of each chicken breast. Close the chicken around the filling and secure with toothpicks.
6. Place the beaten eggs in a wide, shallow bowl.
7. In a separate wide, shallow bowl, stir together the bread crumbs, Parmesan, Italian seasoning, salt, and pepper. Carefully dip each stuffed breast first in the eggs and then into the bread crumb mixture, coating well. Arrange the coated chicken on the prepared rack on the baking sheet.
8. Bake for 35 to 40 minutes, or until the coating is golden brown and the chicken is cooked through and the juices run clear. Serve hot.

Flaky-Crust Chicken and Veggie Potpie

Prep time: 15 minutes | Cook time: 38 minutes | Serves 6

For the Crust:

1¼ cups all-purpose flour, plus more for the work surface
½ teaspoon table salt
8 tablespoons cold, unsalted butter, cut into small pieces
2 to 3 tablespoons ice-cold water

For the Filling:

$^1/_3$ cup unsalted butter
$^1/_3$ cup all-purpose flour, plus more for rolling the dough
$^1/_3$ cup chopped onion
½ teaspoon kosher salt
¼ teaspoon freshly ground black pepper
1¾ cups chicken broth
$^2/_3$ cup milk
2½ to 3 cups cut-up cooked chicken
1 (10-ounce / 283-g) package frozen peas and carrots

Make the Crust

1. In a large bowl, stand mixer, or food processor, combine the flour and salt. Stir or pulse to mix.
2. Add the butter. Using a pastry cutter, two knives, or a mixing blade attachment on your mixer, cut it into the flour until the mixture begins to come together in crumbs.
3. While stirring or with the mixer or food processor running, slowly add the water, 1 tablespoon at a time, until the dough balls up and

begins to pull away from the sides of the bowl. Remove the dough, form it into a ball, and flatten it into a disk. Wrap the disk in plastic wrap and refrigerate for at least 30 minutes.

Make the Filling

4. Select Convection Bake and preheat the oven to 400ºF.

5. In a large skillet over medium heat, melt the butter.

6. Add the flour, onion, salt, and pepper. Cook for 3 minutes, stirring constantly.

7. Add the chicken broth and milk and bring to a boil, continuing to stir constantly. Boil for 1 minute, while stirring, until the mixture thickens.

8. Add the chicken and peas and carrots and stir to combine. Transfer the mixture to a 9-inch pie dish and let cool for several minutes.

9. On a lightly floured work surface, roll the dough into a 10-inch circle. Place it on top of the filling in the pie dish. Poke several holes in the crust with a skewer or make a few slashes with a sharp knife. Fold the crust over and crimp it decoratively around the edge. Bake for about 35 minutes, or until the crust is golden brown and the filling is bubbling.

Turkey Breast Roulade with Sausage Stuffing

Prep time: 15 minutes | Cook time: 1½ hours | Serves 8

Nonstick cooking spray, for preparing the pan
2 tablespoons unsalted butter
1 onion, diced
2 celery stalks, diced
3 garlic cloves, minced
8 ounces (227 g) mild Italian sausage, ground or casings removed
½ cup white wine
1 tablespoon finely chopped fresh thyme leaves
1 large egg, beaten
9 cups dried bread cubes, or cornbread cubes
1¾ cups chicken broth
3 tablespoons chopped fresh flat-leaf parsley leaves
2½ teaspoons kosher salt, divided
1¼ teaspoons freshly ground black pepper, divided
1 (4-pound / 1.8-kg) boneless turkey breast, butterflied (see Preparation tip)
2 tablespoons olive oil, divided

1. Select Bake and preheat the oven to 350ºF (180ºC).

2. Place a roasting rack in a bake pan and spray it with cooking spray. Arrange the oven racks so there is room for the bake pan with the turkey as well as a baking dish containing the extra stuffing.

3. In a large skillet over medium heat, melt the butter.

4. Add the onion and celery. Cook for about 5 minutes, stirring frequently, until softened.

5. Stir in the garlic and sausage. Cook for about 5 minutes more, stirring and breaking up the meat with a spatula, until the sausage is browned.

6. Stir in the white wine and thyme. Cook for 2 minutes more, scraping up any browned bits from the bottom of the pan. Remove from the heat and set aside to cool for a few minutes.

7. In a large bowl, combine the cooled sausage mixture with the egg, bread cubes, chicken broth, parsley, ½ teaspoon of salt, and ¼ teaspoon of pepper, stirring until the bread is fully moistened.

8. Lay a large piece of plastic wrap or parchment paper on your work surface and place the turkey breast on top. Cover the turkey with a second piece of plastic wrap or parchment paper. Using a mallet or rolling pin, pound the meat until it is an even ½ inch thick. Rub the turkey all over with 1 tablespoon of olive oil and season with 1 teaspoon of salt and ½ teaspoon of pepper.

9. Arrange the stuffing mixture in a ½-inch-thick layer over the turkey, leaving a clear 1-inch border all the way around. If you have extra stuffing, place it in a baking dish to bake alongside the turkey roulade. Starting with one of the long sides, roll the turkey around the stuffing into a cylinder. Secure with toothpicks or tie the roll with kitchen twine. Place the turkey roulade seam-side down on the prepared roasting rack. Drizzle with the remaining 1 tablespoon of olive oil and season with the remaining 1 teaspoon of salt and ½ teaspoon of pepper. Bake for about 1 hour, 15 minutes.

10. Add the baking dish with the extra stuffing to the oven after the turkey has been in for about 30 minutes.

11. Use a meat thermometer to test for doneness. The temperature in the middle of the

thickest part of the turkey breast should be at least 155ºF. Remove from the oven, tent loosely with aluminum foil, and let rest for 10 to 15 minutes. To serve, carve into ½-inch-thick pieces.

Orange-Glazed Whole Chicken

Prep time: 5 minutes | Cook time: 1½ hours | Serves 6

1 (3-pound / 1.4-kg) whole chicken, rinsed and patted dry with paper towels

Brushing Mixture:

2 tablespoons orange juice concentrate
1 tablespoon soy sauce
1 tablespoon toasted sesame oil
1 teaspoon ground ginger
Salt and freshly ground black pepper, to taste

1. Preheat the toaster oven to 400ºF (205ºC).
2. Place the chicken, breast side up, in an oiled or nonstick 8½ × 8½ × 2-inch square (cake) pan and brush with the mixture, which has been combined in a small bowl, reserving the remaining mixture. Cover with aluminum foil.
3. Bake for 1 hour and 20 minutes. Uncover and brush the chicken with remaining mixture.
4. Bake, uncovered, for 20 minutes, or until the breast is tender when pierced with a fork and golden brown.

Dijon-Rosemary Chicken Breasts

Prep time: 5 minutes | Cook time: 30 minutes | Serves 2

2 skinless, boneless chicken breast halves

Sauce:

3 tablespoons dry white wine
1 tablespoon Dijon mustard
2 tablespoons nonfat plain yogurt
Salt and freshly ground black pepper, to taste
2 rosemary sprigs

1. Preheat the toaster oven to 400ºF (205ºC).
2. Place each breast on a 12 × 12-inch square of heavy-duty aluminum foil (or regular foil doubled) and turn up the edges of the foil.
3. Mix together the sauce ingredients and spoon over the chicken breasts. Lay a rosemary sprig on each breast. Bring up the edges of the foil and fold to form a sealed packet.
4. Bake for 25 minutes or until juices run clear when the meat is pierced with a fork. Remove the rosemary sprigs.
5. Broil for 5 minutes, or until lightly browned. Replace the sprigs and serve.

Chicken, Vegetable and Rice Casserole

Prep time: 10 minutes | Cook time: 52 minutes | Serves 4

4 skinless, boneless chicken thighs, cut into 1-inch cubes
½ cup brown rice
4 scallions, chopped
1 plum tomato, chopped
1 cup frozen peas
1 cup frozen corn
1 cup peeled and chopped carrots
2 tablespoons chopped fresh parsley
1 teaspoon mustard seed
1 teaspoon dried dill weed
¼ teaspoon celery seed
Salt and freshly ground black pepper, to taste
½ cup finely chopped pecans

1. Preheat the toaster oven to 400ºF (205ºC).
2. Combine all the ingredients, except the pecans, with 2½ cups water in a 1-quart 8½ × 8½ × 4-inch ovenproof baking dish. Adjust the seasonings to taste. Cover with aluminum foil.
3. Bake, covered, for 45 minutes, or until the rice is tender, stirring after 20 minutes to distribute the liquid. When done, uncover and sprinkle the top with the pecans.
4. Broil for 7 minutes, or until the pecans are browned.

Barbecue Turkey Burgers

Prep time: 5 minutes | Cook time: 20 minutes | Serves 4

1 pound (454 g) lean ground turkey breast
2 tablespoons bread crumbs
2 tablespoons barbecue sauce
½ teaspoon garlic powder

½ teaspoon chili powder
Salt and freshly ground black pepper, to taste

1. Combine all ingredients in a bowl, mixing well. Divide into 4 portions and shape into patties.
2. Broil on a rack with a pan underneath for 20 minutes, or until the meat is browned and the juice runs clear when pierced with a fork.

Duck Breast with Asian-Flavored Plums

Prep time: 10 minutes | Cook time: 28 minutes | Serves 4

For the Plums:

1¼ pounds (567 g) plums, halved and pitted
2 tablespoons clear honey
2½ tablespoons light brown sugar
1½ tablespoons soy sauce
2 broad strips of orange zest, plus juice of ½ orange
½ teaspoon ground ginger
½ teaspoon five spice powder
1½ teaspoons crushed red pepper
2 garlic cloves, finely grated
Sea salt flakes and freshly ground black pepper, to taste

For the Duck:

4 duck breasts

1. Preheat the oven to 375ºF (190ºC).
2. Put everything for the plums into a bake pan or ovenproof dish in which the plums can lie in a single layer, seasoning well with salt and pepper. Bake for 15 minutes, then turn the plums over and return to the oven to bake until they have completely collapsed (ripe plums may only need 20 minutes; really hard fruits could take as long as 35 minutes). Mash the cooked plums with a fork and taste for seasoning, then leave to cool.
3. Increase the oven temperature to 400ºF (205ºC).
4. Heat a large ovenproof frying pan and, when it's very hot, put the duck breasts in, skin side down. Cook until the fat starts to run out and the skin is seared and golden, about 3 to 4 minutes. Turn the breasts over and quickly cook them on the other side until colored. Season all over. Put the pan into the oven and roast the duck for 7 minutes.
5. Cut into the underside of a duck breast to see how well it's done: you want them rare—but not raw—in the center (if you don't like them very rare, cook for a little longer until they are the way you like them). Return them to the oven if they're not quite ready, though I wouldn't suggest you roast them for more than 10 minutes in total. When they're done, cover and set aside to rest for about 7 minutes so the juices can "set."
6. Carve the duck into slices and serve with the room-temperature plums.

Chicken and Potato Casserole with Harissa

Prep time: 10 minutes | Cook time: 40 minutes | Serves 4

1 pound (454 g) small waxy potatoes, scrubbed and quartered
2 red onions, halved and cut into wedges
1 head of garlic, cloves separated but not peeled
3 tablespoons extra-virgin olive oil
Sea salt flakes and freshly ground black pepper, to taste
8 good-sized skin-on, bone-in chicken thighs, excess skin neatly trimmed
Finely grated zest of 1 unwaxed lemon, plus juice of ½ lemon
½ to $^{2}/_{3}$ cup Feta cheese, crumbled
$^{2}/_{3}$ cup dill leaves, torn
1 cup Greek yogurt
1 tablespoon harissa

1. Preheat the oven to 400ºF (205ºC).
2. Put the potatoes, onions, garlic cloves, 2 tablespoons of the oil, salt, and pepper into a 12in wide shallow casserole or ovenproof sauté pan. Toss everything around with your hands. Put the chicken thighs on top, skin side up. Brush the remaining oil on the chicken and season it.
3. Bake for 40 to 45 minutes, or until the chicken is golden and the potatoes are tender when pierced with a sharp knife.
4. Squeeze the lemon juice over, then scatter on the zest, Feta, and dill.
5. Put the yogurt into a bowl and spoon the harissa on top. Serve the chicken with the harissa yogurt on the side.

Sherry Chicken and Sweet Potato

Prep time: 20 minutes | Cook time: 45 minutes | Serves 4 to 6

For the Chicken:

8 good-sized skin-on, bone-in chicken thighs, excess skin neatly trimmed
1½ pounds (680.4 g) sweet potatoes, scrubbed and cut into wedges
2½ tablespoons white miso paste
1½ tablespoons clear honey
2 tablespoons sake, or dry sherry
1 tablespoon dark soy sauce
1-inch fresh ginger, peeled and finely grated
3 garlic cloves, finely grated
1 red Fresno chili, halved and finely chopped (use the seeds)
12 to 18 scallions, trimmed
3 teaspoons black or toasted white sesame seeds (or a mixture of both)
Stir-fried green vegetables, to serve

For the Final Basting:

1 tablespoon white miso paste
1 tablespoon clear honey
½ tablespoon dark soy sauce
½ tablespoon sake, or dry sherry

1. Preheat the oven to 400ºF (205ºC).
2. Put the chicken thighs or joints into a big bake pan with the sweet potato wedges (they should be able to lie—more or less—in a single layer).
3. In a small bowl, mix everything else together, except the scallions and sesame seeds. Pour this over the chicken and sweet potatoes, turning everything over so the ingredients get well coated. Finish with the chicken skin side up.
4. Bake for 45 minutes, basting every so often and turning the sweet potato wedges over.
5. Stir the ingredients for the final basting together in another small bowl.
6. About 15 minutes before the end of cooking time, take the pan out of the oven, add the scallions, and pour the final basting mixture over everything. Return to the oven. The scallions should become soft and slightly charred.
7. Transfer the chicken and vegetables to a warmed platter and sprinkle with the sesame seeds. Serve immediately, with stir-fried green vegetables.

Chicken and Plums Casserole

Prep time: 20 minutes | Cook time: 45 minutes | Serves 4

For the Chicken:

8 good-sized, skin-on bone-in chicken thighs, excess skin neatly trimmed
2 teaspoons ground sumac
1 teaspoon ground coriander
4 garlic cloves, finely grated
3 tablespoons extra-virgin olive oil
Sea salt flakes and freshly ground black pepper, to taste
2 red onions, cut into fine crescent moon-shaped slices
8 plums (preferably crimson- fleshed and firm), halved and pitted
¼ cup clear honey
3 tablespoons pomegranate molasses
½ teaspoon cayenne pepper
1½ teaspoons ground cumin
Finely grated zest of ½ orange
4 teaspoons soft light brown sugar
¼ cup orange juice
3 tablespoons pomegranate seeds

For the Pistachio Relish:

2½ tablespoons shelled unsalted pistachio nuts, chopped
1 garlic clove, finely chopped
3 tablespoons chopped cilantro leaves
1 tablespoon extra-virgin olive oil
Lemon juice, to taste

1. Preheat the oven to 375ºF (190ºC).
2. Put the chicken thighs into a 12in ovenproof dish or shallow casserole in which they can all lie in a single layer. Add the sumac, ground coriander, half the garlic, and all the olive oil, and season. Turn everything over with your hands to make sure it's coated, then cover and marinate in the refrigerator for 1 hour, if you have the time. Mix the onions with the chicken and the marinade, then arrange the thighs so they are skin side up. Dot half the plums among the chicken.

3. In a small bowl, stir the honey and pomegranate molasses together with the cayenne pepper, cumin, orange zest, and the remaining garlic. Spoon half of this over the chicken and plums. Sprinkle half the sugar on the plums and season them, then pour the orange juice around.
4. Bake for 25 minutes, then spoon the rest of the honey and pomegranate molasses over the chicken skin. Add the remaining plums and sprinkle them with the remaining sugar. Return to the oven to cook for a final 20 minutes.
5. For the relish, bash the nuts in a mortar with the garlic and some salt. Add the cilantro and bash a bit more to break it all down a bit, not grind it into a paste, then stir in the olive oil and lemon juice. Season to taste, then spoon it over the chicken and scatter with pomegranate seeds.

Chicken and Potato Casserole with Capers

Prep time: 10 minutes | Cook time: 40 minutes | Serves 4

1¼ pounds (567 g) small waxy potatoes, scrubbed and cut into 1-inch chunks
2 onions, cut into crescent moon-shaped wedges
1 head of garlic, cloves separated but not peeled
10 thyme sprigs
2 unwaxed lemons
3 tablespoons extra-virgin olive oil
Sea salt flakes and freshly ground black pepper, to taste
8 good-sized skin-on bone-in chicken thighs, excess skin neatly trimmed
3 tablespoons capers, drained, rinsed, and patted dry

1. Preheat the oven to 400ºF (205ºC).
2. Put the potatoes into a shallow casserole dish 12in across, or a bake pan in which all the vegetables can lie in a single layer. Add the onions, garlic cloves, and thyme. Finely grate the zest of 1 lemon over this and squeeze on the juice of half of it. Cut the other lemon into fine slices (flick out any seeds you see).
3. Add 2 tablespoons of the extra-virgin olive oil to the vegetables and season them. Toss the lemon slices in and turn everything over with your hands.
4. Put the chicken thighs on top, skin side up, and brush them with the remaining olive oil. Season them, too. Make sure no lemon slices are sticking out, as they will burn quickly; they should be tucked under the chicken.
5. Bake in the oven for 30 minutes. Retrieve some of the lemon slices and put them on top of the chicken, so they can turn golden in the last bit of cooking time. Scatter the capers over and return to the oven for a final 10 minutes. Serve immediately.

Chicken and Hot Italian Sausages Casserole

Prep time: 10 minutes | Cook time: 45 minutes | Serves 6 to 8

3 tablespoons extra-virgin olive oil
8 good-sized skin-on. bone-in chicken thighs, excess skin neatly trimmed
1 pound (454 g) good-quality sweet Italian sausages
3 red bell peppers
2 red onions, halved and cut into crescent moon-shaped slices
1 teaspoon crushed red pepper
8 garlic cloves, finely grated
Sea salt flakes and freshly ground black pepper, to taste
2 tablespoons sherry vinegar
Leaves from 1 rosemary sprig, plus 3 whole rosemary sprigs
Olive oil-roasted potatoes, mashed potatoes, or rice pilaf, to serve

1. Preheat the oven to 375ºF (190ºC).
2. Heat half the olive oil in a big, shallow casserole dish in which the thighs can lie in a single layer, or use a heavy bake pan that can go on the stovetop and in the oven. Quickly brown the chicken on both sides, if you don't want to cook it through, just get some color on it. Then remove from the pan. Do the same with the sausages, coloring them all over.
3. Cut the sausages on the diagonal into pieces. Halve and deseed the peppers and cut each half into 4 pieces lengthwise.
4. Toss the peppers and onions into the casserole or bake pan with the crushed red pepper, garlic, seasoning, the rest of the oil, the sherry vinegar, rosemary, and sausages. Turn everything

over with your hands. Put the chicken, skin side up, on top of this.

5. Bake in the oven for 40 to 45 minutes, turning the vegetables over a couple of times. The chicken should be cooked through. Serve either with little potatoes that you've roasted in olive oil, or with mashed potatoes, or rice pilaf (mashed potatoes or rice pilaf scented and colored with saffron would be lovely with this).

Chicken with Vermouth and Mustard

Prep time: 10 minutes | Cook time: 40 minutes | Serves 4

8 good-sized skin-on, bone-in chicken thighs, excess skin neatly trimmed
¼ cup Dijon mustard
1 tablespoon extra-virgin olive oil
Freshly ground black pepper, to taste
½ garlic clove, finely grated
$^{1}/_{3}$ cup crème fraîche
$^{2}/_{3}$ cup dry white vermouth
2 tablespoons very finely chopped flat-leaf parsley leaves
Squeeze of lemon juice
1 tablespoon cold unsalted butter, chopped

1. Preheat the oven to 400ºF (205ºC).
2. Put the chicken thighs into a heavy bake pan in which they can lie in a single layer, sitting snugly together with not much room around them, or into a 12in shallow casserole.
3. In a small bowl, mix the mustard with the olive oil and spread this all over the skin of the chicken. Season with pepper (there's a lot of salt in the Dijon mustard). Mix the garlic with the crème fraîche and dollop it on top of the chicken (it doesn't have to be neat, as it will melt and run off the chicken once it goes into the oven). Pour in about two-thirds of the vermouth at the sides so it runs underneath the chicken.
4. Cook for 40 minutes, adding the rest of the vermouth halfway through.
5. Put the chicken onto a warmed plate and cover it with foil and a couple of tea towels to keep it warm.
6. Quickly bring the juices in the bake pan or casserole to the boil and reduce them a little so they thicken. Add the parsley and lemon juice and whisk in the butter, bit by bit. Return the chicken to the sauce, then serve.

Chicken with Raisin and Bitter Greens

Prep time: 20 minutes | Cook time: 40 minutes | Serves 4

1½ cups sourdough bread, torn into pieces roughly 2in square
1 pound (454 g) small waxy potatoes, scrubbed and cut into chunks
1 large onion, cut into wedges
6 thyme sprigs
2 teaspoons crushed red pepper
1 head of garlic, cloves separated but not peeled
$^{1}/_{3}$ pound (151.2 g) pancetta or slab bacon, in 1 piece
8 good-sized skin-on, bone-in chicken thighs, excess skin neatly trimmed
2 tablespoons sherry vinegar
1 cup amontillado sherry
5 tablespoons extra-virgin olive oil
Sea salt flakes and freshly ground black pepper, to taste
10 thin scallions, trimmed
$^{1}/_{3}$ cup raisins
¼ pound (113.4 g) bitter salad greens (such as radicchio, Belgian endive, frisée, dandelion or treviso)
3 tablespoons toasted pine nuts

1. Preheat the oven to 400ºF (205ºC).
2. Put the bread, potatoes, onion, thyme, crushed red pepper, and garlic cloves into a large bake pan. Cut the pancetta or bacon into ½in chunks and add them to the pan with the chicken. Pour on the sherry vinegar, ¼ cup of the sherry, and 4 tablespoons olive oil. Season and toss everything around with your hands, finishing with the chicken skin side up. Make sure the bread isn't too exposed, or lying at the edges, or it will burn.
3. Bake for 25 minutes, tossing the ingredients around once, but making sure the chicken is still skin side up. Then add another ¼ cup sherry.
4. Mix the scallions in a bowl with the remaining olive oil and add them to the pan, too,

laying them on top of the vegetables. Return to the oven and bake for a final 15 minutes.

5. Pour the remaining sherry into a small saucepan with the raisins and bring to just under a boil. Let sit, then add them to the bake pan 5 minutes before the end of the cooking time.

6. Transfer everything to a large warmed platter or broad, shallow serving dish (unless you're happy to take the bake pan to the table) and mix in whichever of the greens you want to use (or just serve them on the side). Throw on the pine nuts and serve.

Chicken and Veggies with 'Nduja

Prep time: 10 minutes | Cook time: 40 minutes | Serves 4

8 good-sized skin-on, bone-in chicken thighs, excess skin neatly trimmed
1 pound (454 g) head cauliflower, broken into florets
1 pound (454 g) baby waxy potatoes, scrubbed, then halved or quartered, depending on size
2¾ ounces (78 g) 'nduja, broken into nuggets
6 thyme sprigs
3 tablespoons olive oil
Sea salt flakes and freshly ground black pepper, to taste
Green salad, or bitter greens, to serve

1. Preheat the oven to 400ºF (205ºC).

2. Put all the ingredients in a bake pan or a broad, shallow casserole about 12in across, season, and toss around with your hands. The chicken should end up skin-side up. Make sure the nuggets of 'nduja aren't lying on top, or they'll burn.

3. Bake for 40 to 45 minutes, turning everything over about 3 times during the cooking. The 'nduja partly melts and you need to ensure it gets well mixed in.

4. Towards the end of the cooking time, it's good to spoon the bits of 'nduja over the chicken, as it gives it a lovely color. The potatoes should be tender when pierced with a sharp knife and the chicken cooked through. Serve with a green salad or bitter greens.

Chicken with Prunes and Vegetable

Prep time: 20 minutes | Cook time: 45 minutes | Serves 4

2½ tablespoons harissa
1 teaspoon ground turmeric
1 teaspoon ground ginger
½ teaspoon ground cinnamon
1 teaspoon ground cumin
4 garlic cloves, finely grated
1 tablespoon light brown sugar
Sea salt flakes and freshly ground black pepper, to taste
2 tablespoons extra-virgin olive oil
1 pound (454 g) small waxy potatoes, scrubbed
2 onions, sliced
¾ pound (340.2 g) cauliflower florets
About 12 moist prunes (more is fine)
1¼ cups chicken stock
2 preserved lemons, plus 1½ tablespoons brine from the jar
8 good-sized skin-on. bone-in chicken thighs, excess skin neatly trimmed
3 tablespoons roughly chopped cilantro leaves
Greek yogurt, to serve

1. Preheat the oven to 400ºF (205ºC).

2. In a bowl, mix together the harissa, spices, garlic, sugar, salt and pepper, and olive oil.

3. Cut the potatoes into very thin slices and put them into a shallow 12-inch casserole with the onions. Add the cauliflower and prunes. Take one-third of the harissa mixture and toss it with the vegetables. Add the chicken stock and place over medium heat until the mixture is simmering.

4. Remove the flesh from the preserved lemons, keep the rind for scattering on top—chop it, then add it to the rest of the harissa mixture, along with the brine from the jar. Mix the chicken thighs with this mixture, rubbing it all over. Set the chicken on top of the simmering vegetables, skin side up. Season the chicken and put the dish into the oven.

5. Cook for 45 minutes, taking the dish out and scooping the cooking juices up over the chicken a couple of times. You should end up with dark, golden chicken and tender vegetables.

6. Cut the preserved lemon rind into shreds and throw it over the chicken along with the cilantro. Serve with a bowl of Greek yogurt.

Tangy Chicken with Squash and Cauliflower

Prep time: 20 minutes | Cook time: 35 minutes | Serves 4 to 6

1 tablespoon peanut oil
8 good-sized skin-on, bone-in chicken thighs, excess skin neatly trimmed
1 large onion, roughly chopped
4 garlic cloves, finely grated
1¼-inch fresh ginger, peeled and finely grated
2 teaspoons ground coriander
2 teaspoons ground cumin
2 green chilies, halved, seeded, and finely chopped
½ pound (227 g) butternut squash, peeled, seeded, and sliced (prepared weight)
¼ pound (113.4 g) cauliflower florets
1½ cups basmati rice
½ cup chopped cilantro leaves
Finely grated zest and juice of 2 limes
2 Makrut lime leaves
Sea salt flakes and freshly ground black pepper, to taste
1¼ cups coconut milk
$1^2/_3$ cups chicken stock
Chutney and plain yogurt, to serve (optional)

1. Preheat the oven to 375ºF (190ºC).
2. Heat the oil in a shallow casserole or sauté pan 12in in diameter, and quickly fry the chicken thighs just to get some color on them (they will darken further in the oven). Put them on a plate.
3. Sauté the onion in the pan until it's soft and pale gold. Add the garlic, ginger, spices, and chilies and cook for 2 minutes, then stir in the squash and cauliflower. Tip in the rice, half the cilantro, the lime zest, half the lime juice, the lime leaves, and seasoning. Return the chicken to the pan skin side up, along with any juices that have run from it. Season the top of the chicken.
4. Heat the coconut milk and chicken stock in a saucepan until just under boiling. Pour this around the chicken thighs and put the pan into the oven, uncovered. Cook for 35 minutes. The chicken should be cooked through and the liquid should have been absorbed by the rice.
5. Squeeze the remaining lime juice over the top and scatter with the rest of the cilantro. Serve immediately, with chutney and yogurt, if you like.

Chicken, Mushrooms and Pumpkin Rice

Prep time: 15 minutes | Cook time: 45 minutes | Serves 4

For the Chicken and Rice:

½ ounces (14.2 g) dried wild mushrooms
2 cups chicken stock
1 cup basmati rice
1 onion, roughly chopped
¼ pound (113.4 g) cremini mushrooms, trimmed and thickly sliced
8 good-sized skin-on, bone-in chicken thighs, excess skin neatly trimmed
¾ pound (340.2 g) pumpkin or butternut squash, seeded, and chopped into big chunks or wedges (prepared weight)
A little extra-virgin olive oil
Sea salt flakes and freshly ground black pepper, to taste

For the Sage Butter:

5 tablespoons unsalted butter, at room temperature
6 sage leaves, finely chopped
1 small garlic clove, finely grated

1. Preheat the oven to 400ºF (205ºC).
2. Soak the wild mushrooms in $^1/_3$ cup just-boiled water for 15 minutes.
3. To make the sage butter, mash the butter with the sage and garlic and set it aside (I only chill this if I'm going to keep it for a while).
4. Drain the wild mushrooms, adding their soaking liquid to the chicken stock.
5. Wash the rice in a sieve under the cold tap, until the water runs clear, to remove the excess starch.
6. Put the onion and both the cremini and dried mushrooms into a 12in sauté pan or shallow casserole (the width is very important) and sprinkle on the rice (it may not look like much, but it expands, don't worry). Put the chicken thighs, skin side up, and the pumpkin on top. Sprinkle a little olive oil

over the vegetables and chicken and season well. Bring the stock mixture to a boil, then carefully pour it around the chicken thighs.

7. Bake in the oven for 45 minutes, by which time the chicken will be lovely and golden and the stock will have been absorbed. Put pats of the sage butter over the chicken thighs, allow it to melt, then serve.

Persian-Spiced Roasted Chicken

Prep time: 15 minutes | Cook time: 1 hour | Serves 6

For the Spice Mix:

1 tablespoon black peppercorns
1 teaspoon coriander seeds
Seeds from 8 cardamom pods
1 tablespoon edible dried rose petals (optional)
½ teaspoon freshly grated nutmeg
¾ teaspoon ground turmeric

For the Chicken:

4 pound (1.8 kg) whole chicken
5 garlic cloves, finely grated
2 tablespoons extra-virgin olive oil, plus more to rub
Sea salt flakes and freshly ground black pepper, to taste
1¼ cups Greek yogurt
Small bunch of dill, leaves chopped, any thicker stalks discarded
Rice or bulgur wheat, to serve

For the Quick-Pickled Onions:

½ cup white wine vinegar 3 tablespoons granulated sugar
1 red onion, thinly sliced

1. To make the spice mix, put the peppercorns, coriander seeds, cardamom seeds, and rose petals, if using, into a mortar and bash until roughly ground. Add the nutmeg and turmeric.
2. Spatchcock the chicken. Put it in a large bake pan.
3. Mix 4 of the grated garlic cloves with the 2 tablespoons olive oil and some seasoning. Carefully lift the skin on the chicken breast without tearing it, and loosen it so that you can push the garlic and oil paste over the breast. If you can lift the skin enough, push it over the legs, too.
4. Rub 1 tablespoon of the spice mix all over the bird and season. Smear with olive oil and rub that in, too. Cover and put it into the refrigerator to marinate for up to 6 hours, or you can roast it right away. If you're cooking it now, preheat the oven to 400ºF (205ºC). Bake for 1 hour.
5. For the quick-pickled onions, heat the vinegar with 5 tablespoons of water, the sugar, and a pinch of sea salt flakes until the sugar and salt dissolve. Add the onion and remove from the heat. Leave to sit for 1 hour (longer is fine).
6. Stir the reserved grated garlic clove into the yogurt with the dill. Serve the chicken with the pickled onions, yogurt, and a bowl of rice or bulgur wheat.

Oregano Stuffed Chicken with Feta

Prep time: 15 minutes | Cook time: 1¼ hours | Serves 6

4 pound (1.8 kg) whole chicken
½ cup crumbled Feta cheese
¼ pound (113.4 g) tomatoes, chopped
1 cup crusty sourdough bread, torn into small pieces
4 tablespoons extra-virgin olive oil, plus more to drizzle
2 garlic cloves, finely grated
3 teaspoons dried oregano
Sea salt flakes and freshly ground black pepper, to taste
½ teaspoon cayenne pepper
1¼ cups orzo
2 cups boiling chicken stock
1 tablespoon chopped flat-leaf parsley leaves, or chopped leaves from 4 oregano sprigs
Salad greens or roasted bell peppers, to serve

1. Preheat the oven to 400ºF (205ºC).
2. Put the chicken into an ovenproof dish—I use a cast-iron one—which is 12in in diameter. Mix the Feta, tomatoes, bread, olive oil, garlic, half the dried oregano, and some seasoning in a bowl. Stuff this into the chicken cavity.
3. Rub the chicken—breast and legs—with the cayenne, sprinkle with the rest of the dried oregano, then season the bird and drizzle it with olive oil.
4. Bake in the oven for 50 minutes.

5. Sprinkle the orzo around the chicken and pour on the boiling stock. Return to the oven for a final 20 minutes. Check during this time to make sure the orzo isn't becoming dry: there should be enough stock in it, but top it up with a little boiling water if you need to.
6. The chicken should be cooked: check by piercing it deeply between the leg and the body, the juices that run out should be clear, with no traces of pink. The orzo should be tender and the stock should have been absorbed.
7. Stir the fresh chopped herbs into the orzo and serve the chicken right from the dish. Salad greens or roasted red peppers is all you need on the side.

Sweet-Sour Chicken and Sausage with Rice

Prep time: 10 minutes | Cook time: 1¼ hours | Serves 6

4 pound (1.8 kg) whole chicken
10 garlic cloves, finely grated
2 tablespoons dried oregano
1 tablespoon sea salt flakes and lots of freshly ground black pepper
4 tablespoons extra-virgin olive oil
Juice of 2 lemons
3 tablespoons unsalted butter
6 Spanish chorizo cooking sausages
Packed ¾ cup light brown sugar
¼ cup red wine vinegar
Boiled rice, to serve

1. Put the chicken into a dish or a large plastic food storage bag. In a bowl, mix the garlic, oregano, salt, pepper, olive oil, and lemon juice, and rub this inside the chicken as well as outside. Cover the dish, or seal the bag, and leave in the refrigerator overnight, or for at least 1 hour. Bring it to room temperature.
2. Preheat the oven to 400ºF (205ºC).
3. Scrape the marinade off the outside of the bird (or the oregano and garlic will burn) and heat the butter in a casserole dish big enough for the chicken. Brown the chicken, breast side down first, then on the other sides, being careful not to burn it. Take it out and add the sausages to the pan. Brown them all over, then add the sugar and vinegar. Bring to a boil, stirring to help the sugar dissolve, then reduce the heat to low. Push the sausages to the edges of the pan and put the chicken in the middle, breast side down.
4. Transfer to the oven and cook for 20 minutes. Reduce the oven temperature to 375ºF (190ºC), cover, and cook for a further 30 minutes. Spoon the juices up over the bird, turn it breast side up, and bake for a final 15 minutes, uncovered. Check for doneness by piercing the bird between the leg and body: the juices that run out should be clear, with no trace of pink.
5. Slice the sausages and carve the chicken, and give everyone some sausage, some chicken, and plenty of the cooking juices. This really calls for boiled rice on the side.

Garlicky Oregano Chicken with Chipotle Allioli

Prep time: 15 minutes | Cook time: 1 hour | Serves 6

For the Chicken:
4 pound (1.8 kg) whole chicken
10 garlic cloves, finely grated
½ tablespoon sea salt flakes
1 red Fresno chili, halved, seeded, and finely chopped
1½ tablespoons dried oregano
2 tablespoons extra-virgin olive oil
Juice of 1 lemon
Roast sweet potato wedges, to serve (optional)

For the Chipotle Allioli:
1 egg yolk
1 teaspoon Dijon mustard
2 garlic cloves, finely grated
½ cup mixed peanut and extra-virgin olive oils
1 tablespoon chipotle paste
Lemon juice, to taste
Sea salt flakes and freshly ground black pepper, to taste

1. To spatchcock the chicken, set the bird on a work surface, breast side down, legs towards you. Using good kitchen scissors or poultry shears, cut through the flesh and bone along both sides of the backbone. Remove the backbone (you can keep it for stock). Open the chicken, turn it over, then flatten it

by pressing hard on the breastbone with the heel of your hand. You'll feel it breaking and flattening under your hand. Remove any big globules of fat and neaten the ragged bits of skin. Now you have a spatchcocked bird.

2. Put the chicken into a dish that fits in your refrigerator. Mix all the other ingredients to make a marinade. Gently loosen the skin of the breast, pushing your fingers between the skin and flesh. Work your way under the skin down to the legs. Spoon some marinade in here, then spread it over the chicken on both sides. Cover and put into the refrigerator for a few hours if you can, turning it once. Bring the bird to room temperature.

3. Preheat the oven to 400ºF (205ºC). Put the chicken into a bake pan and bake for 1 hour, basting a few times during the cooking.

4. Make the allioli while the chicken is cooking. Mix the egg yolk, mustard, and garlic in a bowl. Using electric beaters or a wooden spoon, gradually add the oils in little drops, making sure each is incorporated before you add the next. If it splits, start again with a new egg yolk and gradually add the curdled mixture. Add the chipotle paste, lemon juice to taste (start with about 1 tablespoon), and seasoning. If you're making this more than 1 hour ahead, cover and keep it in the fridge, stirring it when you take it out. (Don't serve it cold from the refrigerator.)

5. Check to see if the chicken is cooked properly. Cut into pieces and serve with the chipotle allioli. Roasted sweet potato wedges are brilliant with it.

Sumptuous Indian-Spiced Chicken with Coconut

Prep time: 25 minutes | Cook time: 53 minutes | Serves 6

For the Spice Paste:

1 teaspoon black mustard seeds
1 teaspoon black peppercorns
1 tablespoon cumin seeds
1 tablespoon coriander seeds
1 teaspoon garam masala
½ teaspoon ground turmeric
¼ teaspoon ground cinnamon
2 red Fresno chilies, halved and seeded
3 garlic cloves, finely grated
¾-inch fresh ginger, peeled and chopped
2 tablespoons malt vinegar
1 tablespoon peanut oil

For the Chicken:

4 pound (1.8 kg) whole chicken
Sea salt flakes and freshly ground black pepper, to taste
1 tablespoon peanut oil
1 large onion, finely chopped
3 garlic cloves, finely grated
¾-inch fresh ginger, peeled and finely grated
14 ounces (397 g) can of cherry tomatoes in thick juice
1 teaspoon light brown sugar (optional)
14 ounces (397 g) can of coconut cream
1 pound (454 g) sweet potatoes, scrubbed, cut into chunks (peel them if you want to)
½ cup roughly chopped cilantro leaves
Boiled rice, naan bread and raita (optional), to serve

1. Preheat the oven to 400ºF (205ºC).

2. Start by making the spice paste. Put the mustard seeds in a frying pan over medium heat and cook until the seeds start to pop (this happens in less than a minute). Add the peppercorns, cumin and coriander seeds, garam masala, turmeric, and cinnamon. Cook for 2 minutes.

3. Scrape the spice mix into a mini food processor with the chilies, garlic, ginger, malt vinegar, and oil. Process to a paste. If you don't have a mini food processor, put the dry spices into a mortar, add the chilies, garlic, and ginger, and grind to a paste, gradually adding the vinegar and oil. Rub about half the spice paste all over the chicken and season the bird in the cavity and outside.

4. Heat the oil in a casserole dish big enough to hold the chicken. Sauté the onion until soft and golden, then add the garlic, ginger, and the rest of the spice paste and cook for 2 minutes. Add the tomatoes, seasoning, and sugar, if using, and cook for another 4 minutes or so, or until it has reduced a little and isn't quite as sloppy. Add the coconut cream and bring to just under a boil, then put the chicken in with the sweet potatoes, spoon over the juices, and put into the oven, uncovered.

5. Cook for 20 minutes, then cover, reduce the oven temperature to 375ºF (190ºC), and cook for a

further 30 minutes. Spoon the juices over the bird and return it to the oven for a final 15 minutes, uncovered. Check for doneness by piercing the chicken between the leg and the main body: the juices that run out should be clear, with no trace of pink.

6. Scatter the cilantro over everything and serve the chicken from the pot. You'll need boiled rice or naan bread on the side, and maybe some raita.

Spicy-Garlicky Chicken Sandwiches

Prep time: 15 minutes | Cook time: 12 minutes | Serves 4

5 or 6 large garlic cloves
3 tablespoons extra-virgin olive oil, divided
2 (8- to 10-ounce / 227- to 283-g) boneless, skinless chicken breasts
1 teaspoon kosher salt, divided
1 cup all-purpose flour
1 teaspoon Cajun or Creole seasoning
2 large eggs
½ teaspoon hot sauce
2 cups panko bread crumbs
$^{1}/_{3}$ cup mayonnaise
4 ciabatta rolls or other sturdy buns, split in half
Lettuce and tomato slices, for serving (optional)

1. Select Bake and preheat the oven to 400ºF (205ºC). Set a rack in a sheet pan.
2. Put the garlic cloves on a piece of aluminum foil and drizzle with 1 tablespoon of oil. Place in the oven while it preheats.
3. Place the chicken breasts on a cutting board and cut each one in half parallel to the board so that you have four flat fillets. Place a piece of plastic wrap over the chicken pieces and use a rolling pin or small skillet to gently pound them to an even thickness of about ½ inch. Season the chicken on both sides with ½ teaspoon of salt.
4. In a shallow bowl, mix the flour, remaining ½ teaspoon of salt, and the Cajun seasoning. In another shallow bowl, whisk together the eggs and hot sauce. In a third shallow bowl, combine the panko and remaining 2 tablespoons of oil.
5. Lightly dredge both sides of the chicken pieces in the seasoned flour, then dip them in the egg wash to coat completely, letting the excess drip off. Finally, dredge the chicken in the panko. Carefully place the breaded chicken pieces on the prepared rack.
6. Bake the chicken for 7 to 8 minutes, then carefully turn the pieces over. Return the pan to the oven and bake for another 5 to 6 minutes, until the chicken is no longer pink in the center.
7. Let the chicken rest while you make the sauce. Put the mayonnaise in a small bowl. Remove the packet of garlic from the oven and smash it before adding it to the mayonnaise. Smash the garlic and stir to combine.
8. Divide the sauce among the bun bottoms and top each with a piece of chicken. Add lettuce and tomato slices (if using) and close the buns.

Garlic Chicken Thighs with Root Vegetable

Prep time: 10 minutes | Cook time: 30 minutes | Serves 4

¼ cup olive oil
2 pounds (907 g) bone-in, skin-on chicken thighs
1½ teaspoons kosher salt, divided
1 small lemon
20 garlic cloves
12 ounces (340 g) small red potatoes (about 2 inches in diameter), quartered
2 large carrots, peeled and cut into 1-inch pieces
$^{1}/_{3}$ cup low-sodium chicken broth
½ teaspoon freshly ground black pepper

1. Select Bake and preheat the oven to 425ºF (220ºC). Coat a sheet pan with the oil and place in the oven while it preheats.
2. Salt the chicken thighs on both sides with ¾ teaspoon of salt.
3. When the oven is heated, remove the sheet pan and place the chicken thighs skin-side down on it. Bake the chicken for 10 minutes.
4. Meanwhile, cut the ends off the lemon and use a mandoline or knife to slice it very thin. Cut the slices in half and remove any seeds.
5. Transfer the chicken thighs to a cutting board or plate. Put the garlic cloves, carrots, and potatoes on the sheet pan and sprinkle with the remaining ¾ teaspoon of salt. Toss to coat with the

oil, then move the vegetables to the outer edges of the pan. Arrange the lemon slices in the center of the pan in two or three layers and place the chicken thighs on top of them, skin-side up.

6. Bake for 30 to 35 minutes, until the chicken registers 175°F and the carrots and potatoes are golden brown and crisp.

7. Transfer the chicken, carrots, and potatoes to a platter. Add the chicken broth and pepper to the sheet pan and mix with the chicken juices, smashing the garlic slightly as you stir. Pour the sauce around the chicken and vegetables and serve.

Teriyaki Roasted Chicken with Snow Peas

Prep time: 10 minutes | Cook time: 18 minutes | Serves 4

½ cup tamari or other gluten-free soy sauce
3 tablespoons honey
1 tablespoon rice vinegar
1 tablespoon rice wine or dry sherry
2 teaspoons minced fresh ginger
2 garlic cloves, minced
1½ pounds (680.4 g) boneless, skinless chicken thighs
2 teaspoons toasted sesame oil
8 to 12 ounces (227- to 340-g) snow peas

1. Select Bake and preheat the oven to 400ºF (205ºC).

2. In a small bowl, whisk together the tamari, honey, vinegar, rice wine, ginger, and garlic until the honey is dissolved. Set aside 2 tablespoons of the marinade and pour the rest into a zip-top bag. Put the chicken thighs in the bag and seal, squeezing as much air out as possible. Squish the chicken around to coat it completely, then let the chicken marinate for 30 minutes, turning the bag every 10 minutes.

3. Put the snow peas on a sheet pan and toss with the reserved marinade and the oil. Move the peas to the outer edges of the pan.

4. Arrange the chicken in a single layer in the center of the pan.

5. Bake the chicken and peas for 8 minutes. Remove from the oven. Turn the chicken over and stir the peas. Bake for another 10 minutes, or until the chicken is browning in spots and the peas are tender.

Adobo-Style Chicken Thigh and Rice

Prep time: 10 minutes | Cook time: 30 minutes | Serves 4

½ cup white vinegar
¼ cup tamari or other gluten-free soy sauce
6 garlic cloves, lightly smashed
1 teaspoon coarsely ground black pepper
2 dried bay leaves
2 pounds (907 g) boneless, skinless chicken thighs
1 cup long-grain white rice
1¼ cups water
½ cup low-sodium chicken broth

1. In a Dutch oven or other oven-safe pot, combine the vinegar, tamari, garlic, pepper, and bay leaves. Add the chicken, cover, and marinate in the refrigerator for 1 to 3 hours.

2. Select Bake and preheat the oven to 350ºF (180ºC).

3. Add the rice, water, and broth to the pot with the chicken, lifting the chicken pieces up so the rice sinks to the bottom. Place the pot over medium heat and bring the liquid to a simmer.

4. Cover the pot and place it in the oven. Bake for 20 minutes, then stir. The rice should be barely tender, with some liquid remaining in the pot. Return the pot to the oven uncovered, and bake for another 10 minutes or so, until the rice is tender and the chicken is done (cut into the thickest part to be sure no pink remains). Remove the bay leaves and garlic.

5. Spoon the rice onto plates and top with the chicken.

Cheesy Chicken Tenders with Veggie

Prep time: 10 minutes | Cook time: 37 minutes | Serves 4

1½ pounds (680.4 g) chicken tenders
1 teaspoon kosher salt, divided
2 tablespoons unsalted butter
1 small onion, chopped
3 garlic cloves, minced

1 pound (454 g) baby spinach
1 (14-ounce / 397-g) can artichoke hearts, drained
½ cup heavy (whipping) cream
4 ounces (113 g) cream cheese, softened
¼ cup grated Parmesan cheese
1 cup shredded Mozzarella cheese

1. Select Bake and preheat the oven to 350ºF (180ºC).
2. Sprinkle the chicken with ½ teaspoon of salt and set aside.
3. In a large cast-iron or other oven-safe skillet, melt the butter over medium heat. When the butter is foaming, add the onion, sprinkle with the remaining ½ teaspoon of salt, and cook, stirring, for 1 to 2 minutes, until the onion starts to soften. Add the garlic and stir for about 30 seconds. Add the spinach in large handfuls, stirring to wilt. Add the artichoke hearts, stirring them into the spinach. Add the heavy cream and cream cheese and cook until the cream cheese has melted into the vegetables. Stir in the Parmesan.
4. Pat the chicken dry and arrange the tenders in a single layer on top of the spinach mixture. Top with the Mozzarella cheese.
5. Put the skillet in the oven and bake for 35 to 40 minutes, until the cheese is lightly browned on top and the mixture is bubbling.
6. Let cool for 5 to 10 minutes, then serve.

Chicken Pot Pie

Prep time: 10 minutes | Cook time: 30 minutes | Serves 4

4 tablespoons (½ stick) unsalted butter
½ cup chopped onion
¼ cup all-purpose flour
½ teaspoon kosher salt
¼ teaspoon freshly ground black pepper
1¾ cups low-sodium chicken broth
½ cup whole milk
2½ cups shredded cooked chicken
2 cups frozen mixed vegetables, thawed
1 (9-inch) refrigerated piecrust

1. Select Convection Bake and preheat the oven to 425ºF (220ºC).
2. In a large cast-iron skillet, melt the butter over medium heat. Add the onion and cook, stirring, until softened. Stir in the flour, salt, and pepper until well blended. Gradually stir in the broth and milk, and cook, stirring occasionally, until bubbly and thickened, about 5 minutes.
3. Stir in the chicken and mixed vegetables. Remove from the heat. Top with the crust, pressing the dough over the edges of the skillet to seal. Cut 3 or 4 slits into the crust.
4. Put the skillet in the oven and bake for 30 to 40 minutes, until the crust is golden brown and the filling is bubbling. Let stand for 5 minutes before serving.

Barbecue Drumsticks with Vegetable

Prep time: 10 minutes | Cook time: 30 minutes | Serves 4

8 chicken drumsticks
1 teaspoon kosher salt, divided
1 pound (454 g) sweet potatoes, peeled and cut into 1-inch chunks
3 tablespoons vegetable oil, divided
1 cup barbecue sauce, plus more if desired
8 ounces (227 g) green beans, trimmed

1. Select Bake and preheat the oven to 375ºF (190ºC).
2. Season the drumsticks on all sides with ½ teaspoon of salt. Let sit for a few minutes, then blot dry with a paper towel.
3. Put the sweet potato chunks on a sheet pan and drizzle with 2 tablespoons of oil. Move them to one side of the pan.
4. Place the drumsticks on the other side of the pan. Brush all sides of the chicken with half the barbecue sauce.
5. Bake for 15 minutes. Brush the drumsticks with the remaining barbecue sauce. Add the beans to the sweet potatoes and drizzle with the remaining 1 tablespoon of oil. Add the remaining ½ teaspoon of salt, and toss the beans and potatoes together. Bake for another 15 to 20 minutes, until the vegetables are sizzling and browned in spots and the chicken is cooked through.
6. If you like, brush the drumsticks with additional barbecue sauce, and serve with the beans and sweet potatoes on the side.

Perfect Upside-Down Chicken Nachos

Prep time: 10 minutes | Cook time: 34 minutes | Serves

1½ pounds (680.4 g) boneless, skinless chicken thighs
1 teaspoon kosher salt
1¼ cups tomato-based salsa
1 (14-ounce / 397-g) can pinto beans, rinsed and drained
8 ounces (227 g) Monterey Jack cheese, shredded
4 ounces (113 g) tortilla chips, or more as needed
1 medium jalapeño pepper, seeded and minced, or ¼ cup sliced pickled jalapeños (optional)

1. Select Bake and preheat the oven to 350ºF (180ºC).
2. Season the chicken thighs on both sides with the salt, and place the thighs in a single layer in a 9-by-13-inch baking dish. Pour about $^2/_3$ cup of salsa over the chicken. Place the pan in the oven and bake for 20 to 25 minutes, until the chicken is nearly done (if the thickest parts aren't quite done, it's okay—the chicken will cook again).
3. Remove the chicken from the dish and chop or pull the meat into ½-inch pieces, discarding any gristle or fat.
4. Pour the beans into the dish and smash lightly with a potato masher or large fork so they are broken up but not smooth. Return the chicken to the pan, add the remaining salsa, and stir to combine.
5. Increase the oven temperature to 400ºF (205ºC) and place the dish in the oven, don't wait for the temperature to rise. Cook the chicken and beans for 7 to 8 minutes, until bubbling.
6. Sprinkle about one-quarter of the cheese over the chicken mixture. Arrange the tortilla chips over the chicken in an even layer, covering the chicken mixture but not overlapping the chips too much. Sprinkle the remaining cheese over the chips, then top with the jalapeño (if using).
7. Return to the oven and bake for 5 to 7 minutes, until the cheese is melted and the chips are beginning to brown on the edges.
8. Serve immediately, scooping the chicken and beans out with the chips.

Simple Chicken Cordon Bleu

Prep time: 10 minutes | Cook time: 30 minutes | Serves 4

Nonstick cooking spray
2 (10- to 12-ounce / 283- to 340-g) boneless, skinless chicken breasts
½ teaspoon kosher salt
4 teaspoons Dijon mustard
4 thin slices prosciutto
4 thin slices Gruyère, Emmental, or other Swiss-style cheese
$^2/_3$ cup panko bread crumbs (gluten-free if necessary)
2 tablespoons unsalted butter, melted
¼ cup grated Parmesan cheese

1. Select Bake and preheat the oven to 375ºF (190ºC). Spray a 9-by-13-inch baking dish with cooking spray.
2. Lay the chicken breasts flat on a cutting board. With your knife parallel to the board, slice each breast across, for a total of four flat pieces. Sprinkle the chicken with the salt. Lay a piece of plastic wrap over the chicken pieces, and use the heel of your hand to press the chicken into a more even thickness.
3. Transfer the chicken pieces to the prepared baking dish. Spread 1 teaspoon of mustard on each chicken piece. Layer one slice of ham and one slice of cheese evenly over each chicken piece.
4. In a small bowl, mix together the bread crumbs, melted butter, and Parmesan cheese. Sprinkle the mixture over the top of each piece.
5. Bake for 30 to 35 minutes, until the topping is browned and the chicken is done—slide a paring knife into one of the chicken pieces to be sure.

Balsamic Turkey with Carrots and Snap Peas

Prep time: 10 minutes | Cook time: 20 minutes | Serves 4

2 (12-ounce / 340-g) turkey tenderloins
1 teaspoon kosher salt, divided
3 tablespoons balsamic vinegar
2 tablespoons honey
1 tablespoon Dijon mustard
½ teaspoon dried thyme

6 large carrots, peeled and cut into ¼-inch-thick slices
8 ounces (227 g) snap peas
1 tablespoon extra-virgin olive oil
1. Select Bake and preheat the oven to 375ºF (190ºC).
2. If your turkey tenderloins are not pre-brined, sprinkle them with ¾ teaspoon of salt. Place the turkey on a sheet pan.
3. In a small bowl, mix the balsamic vinegar, honey, mustard, and thyme.
4. Put the carrots and snap peas in a medium bowl and drizzle with the oil. Add 1 tablespoon of the balsamic mixture and the remaining ¼ teaspoon of salt, and toss to coat. Scatter the vegetables on the pan around the turkey tenderloins. Brush the tenderloins with about half of the remaining balsamic mixture.
5. Bake the turkey and vegetables for 10 to 12 minutes, then remove the pan from the oven. Gently stir the vegetables. Flip the tenderloins and baste them with the remaining balsamic mixture. Cook for another 10 to 15 minutes, until the center of the tenderloins registers 155ºF (68ºC) on a meat thermometer.
6. Slice the turkey and serve with the vegetables.

Herb Buttery Turkey Breast

Prep time: 10 minutes | Cook time: 35 minutes | Serves 4

1 (4- to 5-pound / 1.8- to 2.3-kg) bone-in turkey breast, split at the breastbone
2½ teaspoons kosher salt, divided
6 tablespoons (¾ stick) unsalted butter, softened, divided
½ small onion, finely chopped
1 celery stalk, finely chopped
½ teaspoon freshly ground black pepper, divided
2 tablespoons finely chopped fresh sage, divided
2 teaspoons finely chopped fresh thyme, divided
¾ cup chicken broth
4 cups stale cornbread, crumbled into large pieces
1 large egg, beaten
1. Select Bake and preheat the oven to 400ºF (205ºC).
2. Sprinkle the turkey breast halves with 1¼ teaspoons of salt. Let it rest while you make the dressing.
3. In a large, oven-safe skillet, melt 3 tablespoons of butter over medium-high heat. Add the onion, celery, remaining 1¼ teaspoons of salt, and ¼ teaspoon of pepper and sauté until the vegetables soften, 5 to 6 minutes. Stir in 1 tablespoon of sage, 1 teaspoon of thyme, and the chicken broth and simmer, uncovered, until the liquid is reduced by about a third, about 3 minutes. Add the cornbread and toss to mix. Stir in the egg.
4. In a small bowl, mix the remaining 3 tablespoons of butter with the remaining 1 tablespoon of sage, 1 teaspoon of thyme, and ¼ teaspoon of pepper. With your fingers, loosen the skin over the turkey breast meat. Scoop half the butter mixture under the skin on each breast half and spread it around with your hands as evenly as possible. Place the turkey breast halves on top of the dressing in the skillet.
5. Transfer the skillet to the oven and bake until a meat thermometer inserted into the turkey reaches 160ºF (71ºC), 35 to 45 minutes. Remove the skillet from the oven and let the turkey rest for 5 to 10 minutes before carving. Serve the turkey with the dressing.

Duck Breast with Potato

Prep time: 5 minutes | Cook time: 12 minutes | Serves 4

2 (1-pound / 454-g) boneless, skin-on duck breast halves
2 teaspoons kosher salt
1 pound (454 g) russet potatoes, peeled and cut into very thin sticks
1. Select Bake and preheat the oven to 400ºF (205ºC). Place a sheet pan in the oven as it heats.
2. With a very sharp knife, gently score the skin side of each duck breast, cutting through the skin and fat but not into the flesh. Space the scores ¼ to ½ inch apart. Turn the breast 90 degrees and score at right angles to the first series of scores. You'll have a diamond pattern of cuts over the skin. Sprinkle both sides with 1 teaspoon of salt.
3. When the oven is up to temperature, take the pan out and arrange the breasts on it, skin-side

down. Bake until the skin is light brown and beginning to crisp and most of the fat has rendered, about 4 minutes.

4. Remove the pan from the oven and arrange the potatoes around the breasts. Toss them to coat with the rendered duck fat and sprinkle with the remaining 1 teaspoon of salt. Bake for another 3 to 4 minutes, until the duck skin is dark golden brown.

5. Turn the breasts over and toss the potatoes. Continue to bake until the duck reaches an internal temperature of 150ºF (66ºC). This can take anywhere from 4 to 8 minutes, depending on the type of duck and the size of the breasts.

6. Remove the pan from the oven and let it rest for 5 minutes before slicing the duck. Serve with the fries.

Marinated Coconut Chicken with Pineapple

Prep time: 10 minutes | Cook time: 20 minutes | Serves 4

2 skinless, boneless chicken breasts, cut into 1 × 3-inch strips
2 tablespoons chopped onion
1 bell pepper, chopped
1 (5-ounce / 142-g) can pineapple chunks, drained
2 tablespoons grated unsweetened coconut

Marinade:

1 teaspoon finely chopped fresh ginger
2 garlic cloves, finely chopped
1 teaspoon toasted sesame oil
1 tablespoon brown sugar
2 tablespoons soy sauce
¾ cup dry white wine

1. Combine the marinade ingredients in a medium bowl and blend well. Add the chicken strips and spoon the mixture over them. Marinate in the refrigerator for at least 1 hour. Remove the strips from the marinade and place in an oiled or nonstick 8½ × 8½ × 2-inch square (cake) pan. Add the onion and pepper and mix well.

2. Broil for 8 minutes. Then remove from the oven and, using tongs, turn the chicken, pepper, and onion pieces. (Spoon the reserved marinade over the pieces, if desired.)

3. Broil again for 8 minutes, or until the chicken, pepper, and onion are cooked through and tender. Add the pineapple chunks and coconut and toss to mix well.

4. Broil for another 4 minutes, or until the coconut is lightly browned.

Sesame Balsamic Chicken Breast

Prep time: 5 minutes | Cook time: 20 minutes | Serves 2

2 skinless, boneless chicken breast filets
3 tablespoons sesame seeds

Mixture:

2 tablespoons sesame oil
2 teaspoons soy sauce
2 teaspoons balsamic vinegar

1. Combine the mixture ingredients in a small bowl and brush the fillets liberally. Reserve the mixture. Place the fillets on a broiling rack with a pan underneath.

2. Broil 15 minutes, or until the meat is tender and the juices, when the meat is pierced, run clear. Remove from the oven and brush the fillets with the remaining mixture. Place the sesame seeds on a plate and press the chicken breast halves into the seeds, coating well.

3. Broil for 5 minutes, or until the sesame seeds are browned.

Chicken Breast in Mango Sauce

Prep time: 10 minutes | Cook time: 40 minutes | Serves 2

2 skinless and boneless chicken breast halves
1 tablespoon capers
1 tablespoon raisins

Mango Mixture:

1 cup mango pieces
1 teaspoon balsamic vinegar
½ teaspoon garlic powder
1 teaspoon fresh ginger, peeled and minced
½ teaspoon soy sauce
½ teaspoon curry powder
1 tablespoon pimientos, minced
Salt and pepper, to taste

1. Preheat the toaster oven to 375ºF (190ºC).
2. Process the mango mixture ingredients in a food processor or blender until smooth. Transfer to an oiled or nonstick 8½ × 8½ × 2-inch square (cake) pan and add the capers, raisins, and pimientos, stirring well to blend. Add the chicken breasts and spoon the mixture over the breasts to coat well.
3. Bake for 40 minutes. Serve the breasts with the sauce.

Tasty Meat and Vegetable Loaf

Prep time: 10 minutes | Cook time: 35 minutes | Serves 4

1 to 1½ pounds (454- to 680.4-g) ground turkey or chicken breast
1 egg
1 tablespoon chopped fresh parsley
2 tablespoons chopped bell pepper
3 tablespoons chopped canned mushrooms
2 tablespoons chopped onion
2 garlic cloves, minced
½ cup multigrain bread crumbs
1 tablespoon Worcestershire sauce
1 tablespoon ketchup
Freshly ground black pepper, to taste

1. Preheat the toaster oven to 400ºF (205ºC).
2. Combine all the ingredients in a large bowl and press into a regular-size 4½ × 8½ × 2¼-inch loaf pan.
3. Bake for 35 minutes, or until browned on top.

CHAPTER 3 MEATS

Chinese-Style Beef and Pepper

Prep time: 15 minutes | Cook time: 16 minutes | Serves 4

1 pound (454 g) sirloin, flat iron, or flank steak, cut into ¼-inch-thick strips
1 teaspoon kosher salt
¼ cup low-sodium beef or chicken broth
¼ cup dry sherry or rice wine
3 tablespoons tamari or other gluten-free soy sauce
3 tablespoons rice vinegar
1 tablespoon toasted sesame oil
1 tablespoon vegetable oil
1 tablespoon sugar
2 teaspoons minced garlic
2 teaspoons minced ginger
1½ teaspoons freshly ground black pepper
1 teaspoon cornstarch
1 medium red bell pepper, cut into bite-size pieces
1 medium green bell pepper, cut into bite-size pieces
1 small onion, cut into ¼-inch-thick wedges
2 scallions, thinly sliced

1. Select Bake and preheat the oven to 375ºF (190ºC).
2. Season the beef slices on all sides with the salt and set aside.
3. In a 9-by-13-inch baking dish, combine the broth, sherry, tamari, vinegar, sesame oil, vegetable oil, sugar, garlic, ginger, black pepper, and cornstarch. Stir to combine.
4. Add the peppers and onion to the baking dish, and toss to coat with the sauce.
5. Bake the vegetables for 6 minutes, or until they're just becoming tender. Add the beef and toss to combine it with the vegetables. Bake for 10 minutes, or until the beef is just cooked through.
6. Serve, garnished with the scallions.

Italian-Style Parmesan Meatloaf

Prep time: 10 minutes | Cook time: 1¼ hours | Serves 4

1 large egg
¼ cup whole milk
24 saltines, crushed but not pulverized
1 pound (454 g) ground chuck
1 pound (454 g) Italian sausage, casing removed
¼ cup grated Parmesan cheese
1 teaspoon kosher salt
1 cup marinara sauce, plus more for serving (optional)
¾ cup shredded Mozzarella cheese

1. Select Bake and preheat the oven to 350ºF (180ºC). Line a sheet pan with aluminum foil.
2. In a large bowl, whisk the egg into the milk, then stir in the crackers. Let sit for 5 minutes to hydrate.
3. With your hands, crumble the ground chuck and sausage into the milk mixture, alternating beef and sausage. When you've added about half the meat, sprinkle about half the grated Parmesan and half the salt over the mixture. Continue breaking up the meat until it's all in the bowl, then add the remaining Parmesan and salt. Gently mix everything together well, but try not to overwork the meat.
4. Form the meat mixture into a loaf shape and transfer the meatloaf to the prepared sheet pan.
5. Bake for 30 minutes, then rotate the pan. Bake for another 20 minutes, then check the temperature. The meatloaf should be 160ºF (71ºC). Cook for another 10 to 20 minutes to reach the desired temperature.
6. When the meatloaf reaches 160ºF (71ºC), increase the oven temperature to 400ºF (205ºC). Spread the marinara sauce over the top of the meatloaf and sprinkle with the Mozzarella. When the oven is up to temperature, return the meatloaf to the oven and bake until the cheese is bubbling and lightly browned, 6 to 8 minutes.
7. Let the meatloaf cool for 15 to 20 minutes to firm it up. Slice and serve with additional marinara (warmed), if you like.

Beef Roast with Vegetable

Prep time: 10 minutes | Cook time: 1½ hours | Serves 4

1 (2½-pound / 1.1-kg) beef chuck (shoulder) roast
1 teaspoon kosher salt
½ teaspoon freshly ground black pepper

1 tablespoon vegetable oil
2 tablespoons tomato paste
½ cup dry red wine
2 cups low-sodium beef broth
1 teaspoon Worcestershire sauce
8 ounces (227 g) boiling onions (about 2 inches in diameter)
4 large carrots, peeled and cut into 2-inch pieces
1 pound (454 g) small red or Yukon Gold potatoes (1 to 2 inches in diameter)

1. Select Bake and preheat the oven to 300ºF (150ºC).
2. Season the roast on all sides with the salt and pepper.
3. Heat the oil in a large Dutch oven over medium heat until it shimmers. Brown the roast on all sides, about 8 minutes total. Transfer the roast to a plate. Add the tomato paste to the pot and cook, stirring, until the paste has darkened slightly, about 1 minute. Add the red wine and bring to a simmer, scraping up the browned bits. Stir in the beef broth and Worcestershire sauce. Place the roast in the liquid.
4. Cover and place the pot in the oven. Bake for 60 to 90 minutes, until the roast is barely tender.
5. Add the onions, carrots, and potatoes and return the pot to the oven, uncovered. Bake for another 30 to 40 minutes, until the vegetables are tender and the beef pulls apart easily with a fork.
6. To serve, slice the beef and place on a platter, surrounded with the vegetables. Pour the sauce over the top.

Slow-Cooked Beef Rib Roast

Prep time: 5 minutes | Cook time: 3 hour | Serves 4

Kosher salt (about ½ teaspoon per pound of meat)
Freshly ground black pepper (about ¼ teaspoon per pound of meat)
1 bone-in rib roast (3 or 4 ribs)

1. Line a sheet pan with paper towels and set a rack on it.
2. Mix the salt and pepper together and rub it all over the roast. Place the roast on the prepared rack and pan, tent it very loosely with aluminum foil, and refrigerate for at least 1 and up to 4 days.
3. Set the oven rack in the lower middle position. Select Bake and preheat the oven to 225ºF (107ºC).
4. Remove the roast from the refrigerator. Examine the Bake for dry spots on either the meat or fat, and trim them off. Remove the paper towels from the sheet pan and set the roast back on the rack, fat-side up. Bake to an internal temperature of 130ºF (54ºC) for medium-rare. This will take about 3 hours, but start checking the temperature at 2½ hours.
5. When the desired internal temperature has been reached, remove the roast from the oven and let it rest for 30 to 60 minutes.
6. Turn the oven temperature to 500ºF (260ºC). Ten minutes before serving, put the roast back in the oven for about 7 minutes (checking at 5 minutes) to brown and crisp the crust. Carve and serve immediately.

Oven Baked Goulash

Prep time: 15 minutes | Cook time: 1½ hour | Serves 4

1 pound (454 g) beef chuck roast, trimmed and cut into 1½-inch pieces
1 teaspoon kosher salt, divided
2 tablespoons vegetable oil, divided
2 medium onions, sliced
2 garlic cloves, minced
¼ cup paprika
2 teaspoons caraway seeds
2 teaspoons dried marjoram or oregano
3 cups low-sodium beef broth
1 (14-ounce / 397-g) can diced tomatoes, drained
12 ounces (340 g) kielbasa or other smoked sausage, cut into 1-inch pieces
2 large carrots, peeled and cut into 1-inch pieces
2 medium red bell peppers, cut into 1-inch pieces
8 ounces (227 g) small red potatoes, quartered
$^{1}/_{3}$ cup sour cream (optional)

1. Select Bake and preheat the oven to 350ºF (180ºC).
2. Sprinkle the beef with ½ teaspoon of salt. In a Dutch oven, heat 1 tablespoon of oil over medium heat until shimmering. Working in batches, add the pieces of beef and sear them on two sides, then transfer to a bowl. Add the remaining 1 tablespoon of oil to the pot, then add the onions and garlic and

sprinkle with the remaining ½ teaspoon of salt. Cook, stirring, until the onions and garlic have softened, about 3 minutes. Add the paprika, caraway, and marjoram and stir to coat the onions. Cook for about 1 minute or until the spices are fragrant.

3. Pour in the beef broth and stir to dissolve the spices. Return the beef to the pot, along with the tomatoes, and bring the mixture to a simmer.

4. Cover and place in the oven. Bake for 60 to 90 minutes, until the meat is just tender.

5. Add the sausage, carrots, bell peppers, and potatoes. Cover and bake for 30 minutes, or until the vegetables are tender.

6. Stir in the sour cream (if using) and serve.

Dijon Barbecue Spareribs

Prep time: 10 minutes | Cook time: 3 hours | Serves 4

1 large rack spareribs
1 teaspoon kosher salt
¼ cup yellow mustard
¼ cup Dijon mustard
2 tablespoons honey
1 tablespoon ketchup (gluten-free if desired)
2 teaspoons Worcestershire sauce
1 teaspoon freshly ground black pepper

1. Select Bake and preheat the oven to 250°F. Line a sheet pan with aluminum foil and set a rack in it.

2. Season the ribs on both sides with the salt and place it on the prepared rack and pan.

3. Bake the ribs for 20 minutes. Flip and rotate the ribs, then return them to the oven. Reduce the oven temperature to 225ºF (107ºC).

4. Bake for 2½ to 3 more hours, flipping and rotating every 40 minutes. The ribs are done when the rack of ribs is flexible and the meat has drawn back from the ends of the bones by about ¾ inch.

5. When the ribs are nearly done, make the sauce. In a small saucepan, stir together the mustards, honey, ketchup, Worcestershire sauce, and pepper. Bring to a simmer over medium heat and cook, stirring occasionally, for 15 to 20 minutes, until slightly thickened.

6. When the ribs are done, baste them on the meaty side with some of the mustard sauce and return them to the oven for 5 to 10 minutes to set the sauce.

7. Slice into individual ribs and serve with the remaining sauce.

Bacon-Wrapped Pork with Honey Apple

Prep time: 10 minutes | Cook time: 24 minutes | Serves 4

1 (1- to 1¼-pound / 454- to 567-g) pork tenderloin
1 teaspoon kosher salt, divided
4 to 6 bacon slices (not thick-cut)
2 tablespoons apple cider vinegar
2 tablespoons honey
1 tablespoon Dijon mustard
1 tablespoon olive oil
½ teaspoon dried thyme
1 large apple, peeled, cored, and cut into ¼-inch-thick slices
1 medium onion, cut into ¼-inch-thick slices

1. Select Bake and preheat the oven to 375ºF (190ºC).

2. Sprinkle the pork all over with ¾ teaspoon of salt (if your tenderloin is brined, omit this step). Wrap the tenderloin with the bacon slices, securing the bacon with toothpicks if necessary.

3. In a small bowl, mix together the vinegar, honey, mustard, oil, and thyme.

4. Put the apple and onion slices on a sheet pan. Drizzle with half the honey mixture and toss to coat. Move the apples and onions to the outer edges of the pan. Place the pork in the center of the pan and baste it with about half the remaining honey mixture and sprinkle with the remaining ¼ teaspoon of salt.

5. Bake for 12 minutes. Stir the apples and onions. Turn the tenderloin over and baste with the remaining honey mixture.

6. Return the pan to the oven and bake for another 12 to 15 minutes, until the apples are soft and the interior of the pork registers between 140ºF (60ºC) and 145ºF (63ºC).

Sweet and Sour Pork with Pineapple

Prep time: 15 minutes | Cook time: 16 minutes | Serves 4

1 (1- to 1¼-pound / 454- to 567-g) pork tenderloin, cut into 1-inch pieces
1 teaspoon kosher salt
$^{1}/_{3}$ cup low-sodium chicken broth
2 tablespoons tamari or other gluten-free soy sauce
2 tablespoons ketchup (gluten-free, if desired)
2 tablespoons brown sugar
2 tablespoons rice vinegar
1 tablespoon toasted sesame oil
1 teaspoon cornstarch
1 teaspoon grated ginger
1 red bell pepper, cut into 1-inch pieces
1 green bell pepper, cut into 1-inch pieces
6 scallions, white parts cut into ½-inch pieces, and green parts thinly sliced
1 cup fresh or canned pineapple chunks, drained

1. Select Bake and preheat the oven to 375ºF (190ºC).
2. Sprinkle the pork with the salt and set aside.
3. In a 9-by-13-inch baking pan, combine the chicken broth, tamari, ketchup, brown sugar, vinegar, oil, cornstarch, and ginger. Stir to combine.
4. Add the bell peppers and scallion whites and toss to coat with the sauce.
5. Bake the vegetables for 6 minutes. Add the pork and pineapple and gently stir to combine.
6. Bake for 10 minutes, or until the vegetables are tender and the pork is cooked through. Serve, garnished with the scallion greens.

Curried Lamb

Prep time: 10 minutes | Cook time: 40 minutes | Serves 4

1 pound (454 g) lean lamb for stewing, trimmed and cut into 1 × 1-inch pieces
1 small onion, chopped
3 garlic cloves, minced
2 plum tomatoes, chopped
½ cup dry white wine
2 tablespoons curry powder
Salt and cayenne, to taste

1. Preheat the toaster oven to 400ºF (205ºC).
2. Combine all the ingredients in an 8½ × 8½ × 4-inch ovenproof baking dish. Adjust the seasonings.
3. Bake, covered, for 40 minutes, or until the meat is tender and the onion is cooked.

Lime Lamb and Tomato Kebabs

Prep time: 10 minutes | Cook time: 16 minutes | Serves 4

1 pound (454 g) boneless lean lamb, trimmed and cut into 1 × 1-inch pieces
2 plum tomatoes, cut into 2 × 2-inch pieces
1 bell pepper, cut into 2 × 2-inch pieces
1 small onion, cut into 2 × 2-inch pieces

Brushing Mixture:

¼ cup lime juice
½ teaspoon soy sauce
1 tablespoon honey
1½ teaspoon ground cumin

1. Skewer alternating pieces of lamb, tomato, pepper, and onion on four 9-inch skewers.
2. Combine the brushing mixture ingredients in a small bowl and brush on the kebabs. Place the skewers on a broiling rack with a pan underneath.
3. Broil for 8 minutes. Turn the skewers, brush the kebabs with the mixture, and broil for 8 minutes, or until the meat and vegetables are cooked and browned.

Beef and Vegetable Stew with Beer

Prep time: 10 minutes | Cook time: 50 minutes | Serves 4

1½ cups dark beer
4 tablespoons unbleached flour
2 cups lean top round steak, cut into 1-inch cubes
1 cup peeled and coarsely chopped carrots
1 cup peeled and coarsely chopped potatoes
½ cup coarsely chopped onion
1 cup fresh or frozen peas
2 plum tomatoes, chopped
3 garlic cloves, minced
3 bay leaves
¼ teaspoon ground cumin
Salt and butcher's pepper, to taste

1. Preheat the toaster oven to 400ºF (205ºC).
2. Whisk together the beer and flour in a 1-quart 8½ × 8½ × 4-inch ovenproof baking dish. Add

all the other ingredients and seasonings and mix well, adjusting the seasonings to taste. Cover the dish with aluminum foil.

3. Bake, covered, for 50 minutes, or until the meat is cooked and the vegetables are tender. Remove the bay leaves before serving.

Pork, Veggie and Rice Casserole

Prep time: 10 minutes | Cook time: 45 minutes | Serves 4

2 (6-ounce / 170-g) very lean boneless pork chops, cut into 1-inch cubes
½ cup brown rice
1 cup chunky tomato sauce
½ cup dry white wine
3 tablespoons finely chopped onion
2 small zucchini squashes, finely chopped
2 plum tomatoes, chopped
½ teaspoon ground cumin
½ teaspoon ground ginger
1 teaspoon garlic powder
2 bay leaves
Salt and freshly ground black pepper, to taste

1. Preheat the toaster oven to 400ºF (205ºC).
2. Combine all the ingredients in a 1-quart 8½ × 8½ × 4-inch ovenproof baking dish. Cover with aluminum foil.
3. Bake, covered, for 45 minutes, or until the rice is cooked to your preference. Discard the bay leaves before serving.

Maple Sausages, Apple and Blackberry

Prep time: 15 minutes | Cook time: 40 minutes | Serves 4

8 good-quality chunky pork sausages
2 tart apples, halved (no need to peel or core)
2 medium onions, each cut into 6–8 wedges
2 rosemary sprigs
3½ tablespoons maple syrup
1½ tablespoons Dijon mustard
1 tablespoon extra-virgin olive oil
2 garlic cloves, crushed
Sea salt flakes and freshly ground black pepper, to taste
$^{2}/_{3}$ cup chicken stock
6 ounces (170 g) blackberries
Mashed or baked potatoes, to serve

1. Preheat the oven to 400ºF (205ºC).
2. Tumble the sausages, apples, onions, and rosemary into a heavy flameproof bake pan, shallow casserole, or ovenproof frying pan about 12in across, in which the ingredients can lie snugly in a single layer. There shouldn't be a lot of room around the ingredients or the juices will reduce and burn.
3. In a small bowl, stir together the maple syrup, mustard, olive oil, and garlic, then pour this mixture into the pan. Season and turn the ingredients to coat them. Bake for 40 to 50 minutes, turning over the sausages once. They should be dark and glossy, with the apples completely soft.
4. Remove the dish or pan from the oven and place over medium-high heat, pouring in the stock. Bring almost to a boil, stirring to help the maple syrup and mustard mixture melt into the stock. Add the blackberries to heat through (don't stir from now on, or they will break up) and serve with mashed or baked potatoes.

Cheddar Toad in the Hole

Prep time: 10 minutes | Cook time: 42 minutes | Serves 4

3 extra-large eggs
generous 1 cup all-purpose flour, sifted
½ cup whole milk
½ cup beer
1 tablespoon English mustard
Sea salt flakes and freshly ground black pepper, to taste
3 tablespoons beef fat, or 2 tablespoons peanut oil
8 good-quality pork sausages
24 scallions (not too thin), trimmed
Scant 1 cup coarsely grated Cheddar cheese,

1. Beat the eggs with electric beaters until they're foamy and thick. Add the flour, then the milk and beer alternately, beating on a low speed, until everything is incorporated and the batter is smooth. Add the mustard and season well. Cover and leave to sit for 30 minutes.
2. Preheat the oven to 400ºF (205ºC). Put half the beef fat or oil in a heavy bake pan (the one I use measures 11½ x 9in) and melt it over medium heat.

Add the sausages, turn them over in the fat, then bake for 10 minutes. Now add the scallions, turn both them and the sausages over in the fat, and bake for another 8 minutes. Remove the scallions and sausages from the bake pan.

3. Increase the oven temperature to 425ºF (220ºC). Put the rest of the beef fat or oil in the pan and, when the oven has reached the new hotter temperature, heat it until smoking.

4. Carefully remove the pan from the oven. Return the scallions to it, pour the batter on top, then return the sausages. Bake for another 20 minutes.

5. Take the bake pan out, sprinkle on the cheese, and return to the oven for a final 5 minutes. The batter should be puffed up and golden. Eat immediately.

Herb Buttery Lamb with Vegetable

Prep time: 15 minutes | Cook time: 50 minutes | Serves 4

For the Herb Butter:

5½ tablespoons unsalted butter, at room temperature

3 tablespoons chopped chervil or equal parts flat-leaf parsley leaves mixed with chives

Sea salt flakes and freshly ground black pepper, to taste

1 tablespoon dry white vermouth

For the Lamb and Vegetables:

1 pound (454 g) frozen peas

2 tablespoons unsalted butter

3 tablespoons extra-virgin olive oil

$^{2}/_{3}$ cup dry white vermouth

10 thin scallions, trimmed

$^{2}/_{3}$ pound (302.4 g) radishes, halved lengthways

2 (8-ounce/ 227-g) boneless lamb loin pieces, trimmed

Squeeze of lemon juice

Handful of mint leaves, torn

1. Preheat the oven to 400ºF (205ºC).

2. To make the butter, just mash it with the herbs and seasoning, then slowly mash in the vermouth. You can put this in the refrigerator if you're making it in advance, otherwise it's fine to leave it at room temperature.

3. Put the peas into a 12in shallow casserole or sauté pan with the regular butter (not the herb butter), 1 tablespoon of the olive oil, the vermouth, and some seasoning. Cook in the oven for 25 minutes. After 10 minutes, toss the scallions and radishes in another 1 tablespoon of the oil and season. Stir the peas, then throw the scallions and radishes on top and return to the oven for their final 15 minutes.

4. Season the lamb with pepper and heat the last tablespoon of oil in an ovenproof frying pan over very high heat. Brown the fillets all over, then transfer them to the oven for 10 minutes. Take them out, cover with foil, and keep warm while letting the meat rest for 10 minutes.

5. Squeeze some lemon juice into the peas and radishes and add the mint leaves. Slice the lamb and serve it with the peas and radishes.

Paprika Chops with Beets and Apple

Prep time: 20 minutes | Cook time: 30 minutes | Serves 4

For the Pork:

4 garlic cloves, finely grated

Sea salt flakes

4 teaspoons caraway seeds

2 tablespoons extra-virgin olive oil

4 ($^{2}/_{3}$-pound / 302.4-g) thick pork chops, on the bone

For the Vegetables:

Generous 1 pound (454 g) cooked beets, peeled and quartered

2 medium-sized tart apples, halved, cored and each cut into 12 wedges

2 onions, halved and sliced about ½in thick

3 tablespoons extra-virgin olive oil

¼ cup cider vinegar

1½ tablespoons soft light brown sugar

1 tablespoon Hungarian sweet paprika

¼ teaspoon crushed red pepper

Sea salt flakes and freshly ground black pepper, to taste

To Serve:

Sour cream

Chopped dill (any thick stalks discarded)

1. Put the garlic into a mortar with the salt and caraway seeds and pound with the pestle. Add the olive oil, working it in until you have a rough paste. Put the pork chops in a bowl and add the mixture from the mortar, turning the chops over in it. Cover and marinate in the refrigerator for a while (at least 1 hour if possible, though longer is fine).
2. Preheat the oven to 375ºF (190ºC).
3. Put everything for the vegetables into a gratin dish or a bake pan in which the beets and apples can lie in a single layer. Toss around with your hands and bake in the oven for 10 minutes.
4. Heat a frying or grill pan over high heat until very hot. Add the chops and color them on both sides, as well as on the fat (hold the chops on their sides, gripping them with tongs, so you can color the fat). Season with pepper and a little more salt.
5. Put the chops on top of the vegetables and pour over the cooking juices from the frying pan. Bake for a final 20 minutes; the meat should be cooked through but still tender.
6. Transfer to a warmed serving dish, or serve in the dish in which it was cooked. Spoon some sour cream scattered with dill over the vegetables, or just serve it on the side.

Cheesy Roast Lamb Chops with Veggie

Prep time: 10 minutes | Cook time: 45 minutes | Serves 4

8 thick loin lamb chops
4 tablespoons extra-virgin olive oil, plus a little more
Leaves from 5 thyme sprigs, plus 3 whole thyme sprigs
1 pound (454 g) small waxy potatoes, scrubbed, halved or quartered, depending on size
¾ pound (340.2 g) cherry tomatoes
1 large red onion, cut into wedges
Sea salt flakes and freshly ground black pepper, to taste
1 head of garlic
Scant 1 cup good-quality black olives, pitted or not, as you prefer
5½ ounces goat cheese, broken into rough chunks

1. Put the chops in a dish with 2 tablespoons of the olive oil and half the thyme. Cover and leave to marinate for at least 1 hour, or in the refrigerator overnight.
2. When you're ready to cook, preheat the oven to 400ºF (205ºC).
3. Put the potatoes, along with the tomatoes and onion, into a large gratin dish or a shallow casserole (about 12in across is ideal) in which all the vegetables can lie in a single layer. Add the rest of the oil, some salt and pepper, and the rest of the thyme. Separate the cloves of garlic and add those, too (you don't need to peel them). Toss everything together and bake in the oven for 25 minutes. Add the olives and scatter the goat cheese over the top. Spoon on a little more oil. Return the dish to the oven for 10 minutes.
4. Heat a frying pan over a very high heat until really hot, season the chops, and sear them until browned, about 1½ minutes on each side.
5. Put the chops on top of the vegetables and bake for a final 10 minutes, by which time they should be cooked through, but remain a little rare. The vegetables should be tender and the goat cheese toasted on top.

Pork with Scallion Salad and Korean Dipping

Prep time: 15 minutes | Cook time: 1½ hours | Serves 4

For the Pork and Sauce:

2½ pounds (1.1 kg) boneless 1-inch thick pork belly slices
A little peanut oil
Sea salt flakes and freshly ground black pepper, to taste
3 tablespoons doenjang soy bean paste
2 tablespoons gochujang chili paste
2 tablespoons toasted sesame oil
2 tablespoons maple syrup or clear honey
2 garlic cloves, finely grated
Carrot and cucumber sticks and crisp lettuce, to serve

For the Salad:

3 tablespoons soy sauce
2 teaspoons light brown sugar
2 tablespoons toasted sesame oil

½ teaspoon gochugaru (Korean red pepper powder), or ½ teaspoon crushed red pepper
10 thin scallions, trimmed
1 teaspoon sesame seeds

1. Preheat the oven to 350ºF (180ºC).
2. Dry the pork belly slices with paper towels, if they're damp they won't brown. Then put into a bake pan large enough for them to lie in a single layer. Brush with oil, season, and cook for about 90 minutes, turning the pork over twice during the cooking time and pouring off the excess fat. When they're ready, they should be meltingly tender and golden brown, but sometimes, depending on your oven, they will need a quick blast at 425ºF (220ºC), just until they turn a good color.
3. To make the dipping sauce, stir both the pastes together in a small bowl with the sesame oil, maple syrup or honey, and garlic. Set aside.
4. For the salad, stir the soy sauce and sugar together in a small salad bowl until the sugar has dissolved, then mix in the sesame oil and red pepper powder or crushed red pepper to make a dressing.
5. Soak the scallions in cold water for 5 minutes, then drain and dry. Halve them horizontally, then shred them lengthwise, so that you end up with very fine slices. Toss the soy-sauce dressing with the scallions and sprinkle the sesame seeds on top.
6. Serve the meat with the dipping sauce, the scallion salad, and crispy vegetables: raw carrot and cucumber sticks are good, as well as lettuce leaves

Lamb and Veggie with Mojo Verde

Prep time: 15 minutes | Cook time: 41 minutes | Serves 4

For the Lamb and Vegetables:

8 thick loin lamb chops
1 teaspoon ground cumin
Sea salt flakes and freshly ground black pepper, to taste
5 tablespoons extra-virgin olive oil
1½ pounds (680 g) sweet potatoes, peeled, or scrubbed and unpeeled, as you prefer, cut into chunks
2 medium onions, cut into slim wedges
2 red bell peppers, halved, seeded, and cut into broad strips

For the Mojo Verde:

3 garlic cloves, chopped
1 green bell pepper, halved, seeded, and chopped
5 tablespoons extra-virgin olive oil
2 tablespoons white wine vinegar
1 teaspoon ground cumin
8 cups cilantro leaves

1. Put the lamb chops in a dish—or in a plastic food storage bag—with the cumin, some seasoning, and half the olive oil. Cover (or seal) and put in the refrigerator while you get on with everything else.
2. Preheat the oven to 375ºF (190ºC).
3. Put the sweet potatoes, onions, and peppers into a bake pan in which they can lie more or less in a single layer. Season and add the remaining oil. Toss the vegetables and bake for 30 minutes, turning them once during that time.
4. To make the mojo verde, put everything in a food processor and blitz. (You will have to push the ingredients down the sides of the bowl a couple of times.) Taste for seasoning.
5. Heat a frying pan over high heat until really hot, then sear the chops until browned, about 1½ minutes on each side.
6. Take the bake pan out of the oven and put the chops on top of the vegetables. Return to the oven and cook for a final 10 minutes, by which time the chops should be cooked through, but remain a little rare.
7. Serve the lamb chops and vegetables with the mojo verde.

Soy-Ginger Buttery Steak

Prep time: 10 minutes | Cook time: 15 minutes | Serves 4

For the Butter:

7 tablespoons unsalted butter, at room temperature
4 scallions, trimmed and finely chopped
½-inch fresh ginger, peeled and finely grated
2 tablespoons soy sauce

For the Steak:

Peanut oil, or beef fat, if you have it
4 (½ pound / 227g) sirloin steaks, each about 1¼in thick

Sea salt flakes and freshly ground black pepper, to taste

1. Mash the butter with the scallions, ginger, and soy sauce, gradually working in the soy sauce until amalgamated. You can leave this at room temperature or put it in the refrigerator. Some people like to chill the butter a little, then shape it into a log and wrap it in greaseproof paper, so you can cut it into rounds.
2. Preheat the oven to 300ºF (150ºC). Put in an empty bake pan or metal baking sheet to heat up, large enough to hold all the steaks.
3. Heat 1 large frying pan for 7 to 10 minutes. Add a tiny bit of oil or beef fat. Once it smokes, it is ready.
4. Put the steaks into the pan. First hold the fat of each of them against the bottom of the pan to render it a little and add color, you need to grip each steak with tongs as you do this. Then lay the steaks flat and press down with your tongs. Season and flip the steaks frequently, moving them round the pan and making sure you can hear them sizzle. If the pan gets too hot and the steak is becoming too dark, reduce the heat (you want a good color, but not burned meat).
5. Once the surfaces are well colored (this should take about 4 minutes) transfer the steaks to the hot bake pan or baking sheet in the oven. Finish cooking the steaks in the oven: 2 minutes for rare, 5 minutes for medium-rare.
6. Serve the steaks with a pat of the soy-ginger butter melting over the top.

Pork with Crushed Grapes and Marsala

Prep time: 10 minutes | Cook time: 1½ hours | Serves 6

4 pound (1.8 kg) boned pork loin, rolled and tied
6 garlic cloves, cut into fine slivers
½ tablespoon sea salt flakes
½ tablespoon black peppercorns
Leaves from 3 rosemary sprigs
1 tablespoon juniper berries
2 tablespoons extra-virgin olive oil
1 pound (454 g) black seedless grapes
1½ cups dry Marsala

1. Unroll the pork and lay it on a board, flesh side up. Make incisions all over the meat with a sharp knife, then push the slivers of garlic into the incisions.
2. Crush the salt, peppercorns, rosemary leaves, and juniper berries roughly in a mortar, then stir in the olive oil.
3. Rub the seasoning mix into the pork, again on the flesh side, pushing bits inside the incisions. Put the pork in a dish, cover, and refrigerate overnight.
4. The next day, remove the pork from the refrigerator and allow it to come to room temperature. Preheat the oven to 400ºF (205ºC).
5. Roll the loin firmly, keeping as much of the seasoning inside as you can, then tie it at intervals with kitchen string. Put it in a heavy bake pan and season all over. Bake for 25 minutes, then reduce the oven temperature to 375ºF (190ºC).
6. Pull half the grapes from their stems, cut the rest of the bunch into sprigs, and add them all to the bake pan with 1 cup of the Marsala. Continue roasting for 60 minutes. Test the meat for doneness: the juices should run clear when the flesh is pierced to the center with a metal skewer.
7. Remove the pork from the pan, along with the grapes that are on sprigs, and put them on a warmed serving platter. Cover and allow to rest for 15 minutes.
8. Set the bake pan over medium heat, add the remaining Marsala, and crush the loose grapes into the juices. Boil until you have a slightly syrupy mixture. Serve the pork with the Marsala sauce and the sprigs of roasted grapes.

Beef with Greens and Blue Cheese

Prep time: 15 minutes | Cook time: 30 minutes | Serves 8

For the Beef:

4 pound (1.8 kg) beef tenderloin
Sea salt flakes and freshly ground black pepper, to taste
1 tablespoon peanut oil, olive oil, or beef fat

For the Salad:

1 cup buttermilk
3 tablespoons sour cream

2 tablespoons extra-virgin olive oil
2 tablespoons white balsamic vinegar
1 teaspoon Dijon mustard
1 small garlic clove, finely grated
1 pound (454 g) red bitter greens, a mixture of Treviso (the one that looks like purple quills), radicchio and red Belgian endive is ideal
$^{2}/_{3}$ cup walnuts, lightly toasted
$^{1}/_{3}$ cup crumbled Cashel Blue cheese

1. Preheat the oven to 425ºF (220ºC).
2. Bring the meat to room temperature. Season the beef really well all over and heat the oil or beef fat in a large frying pan. When the fat is smoking, add the beef and brown it on all sides. Transfer the roas to a bake pan and bake for 10 minutes, then reduce the oven temperature to 400ºF (205ºC)) and cook for another 20 minutes. Cover the meat with foil, insulate it with kitchen towels or old towels, and leave it to rest for 15 minutes.
3. To make the dressing, put the buttermilk, sour cream, olive oil, white balsamic vinegar, mustard, garlic, and seasoning into a bowl and mix with a fork. Taste for seasoning.
4. Put the greens into a broad, shallow bowl or onto a platter and throw on the walnuts and the cheese. Drizzle or spoon the dressing over the top (don't drown the leaves, just serve the extra dressing on the side).
5. Slice the beef and serve it with the greens, cheese, and dressing.

Hoisin Pork Butt with Veggies Salad

Prep time: 20 minutes | Cook time:minutes | Serves 6

For the Pork:

4½ pounds (2 kg) boned pork butt
½ cup soy sauce
½ cup clear honey
½ cup hoisin sauce
½ cup amontillado sherry
2 teaspoons five spice powder
1¼-inch fresh ginger, peeled and finely grated

To Serve:

Boiled rice, or soft white bread rolls
Radish and Cucumber Salad, to serve
Crisp lettuce leaves

For the Salad:

3 tablespoons unseasoned rice vinegar
3 teaspoons superfine sugar
Pinch of fine sea salt
¾-inch fresh ginger, peeled and finely grated
1 large garlic clove, very finely chopped or grated
1 cucumber, chilled
$^{2}/_{3}$ pound (302.4 g) radishes (a mixture of colors if possible), quartered, or cut into eighths if they're big
1 teaspoon toasted sesame oil
1 teaspoon toasted sesame seeds (a mixture of white and black, if you like)

1. Remove the skin from the pork and discard. Leave the fat on.
2. Mix together all the other ingredients for the pork in a small bowl to make a marinade. Put this with the pork in a large plastic food storage bag, if possible, or a bake pan. Marinate in the refrigerator for 24 to 48 hours, turning the meat over every so often.
3. Bring the pork to room temperature by removing it from the refrigerator for at least 1 hour before you are going to cook it.
4. Preheat the oven to 275ºF (135ºC).
5. Put the pork into a bake pan in which it will fit snugly (if there is a lot of room around it, the juices and the marinade will just run off and burn) and pour the marinade into a saucepan. Bake the pork for 4½ to 5 hours, or until the meat is soft and melting. Bring the marinade to a boil, then remove from the heat (it's very important to reheat the marinade to the boiling point, so it's safe for you to use it to baste the partly-cooked pork).
6. Now ladle some of the marinade over the pork and return to the oven. Keep adding more of the marinade and basting the pork every 10 minutes for the next hour. Turn it over every time you do this. The pork should end up dark and glossy. If the roast starts to get too dark on the outside, cover it with foil.
7. To make the salad, mix the vinegar, sugar, salt, ginger, and garlic together. Peel the cucumber in stripes. Halve it along its length and scoop out the seeds, then cut it into 1½in lengths. Bash these with a mallet or a rolling pin. Put the cucumber into a serving bowl with the dressing and place in the refrigerator for 20 minutes. When you're ready to eat,

add the radishes and the sesame oil and toss everything together. Scatter the sesame seeds on top.

8. Serve the pork with boiled rice, or in soft white bread rolls, with the radish and cucumber salad, and with crisp lettuce leaves.

Lamb Leg with Root Vegetable

Prep time: 10 minutes | Cook time: 1 hour | Serves 6 to 8

2¼ cups finely grated pecorino cheese
6 garlic cloves, finely grated
Sea salt flakes and freshly ground black pepper, to taste
3 tablespoons extra-virgin olive oil, plus more if needed
$^{1}/_{3}$ cup basil leaves, plus more to serve (optional)
4 pound (1.8 kg) leg of lamb
2 medium red onions, cut into wedges
$1^{1}/_{3}$ pounds (604.8 g) small waxy potatoes, scrubbed, then halved or quartered, depending on size
¾ pound (340.2 g) red and yellow cherry tomatoes, halved or quartered
Generous 1 cup white wine

1. Preheat the oven to 450ºF (235ºC).
2. Put the cheese, garlic, and some salt into a mortar and pound to a rough purée, gradually adding the olive oil. Tear the basil leaves, add them to the mortar, and pound them, too.
3. Place the leg of lamb in a bake pan. Make deep incisions all over it and push the paste from the mortar down into them. You can also loosen the meat around the bone to make a pocket and push the paste into that, too. Season all over and put into the oven.
4. Bake for 15 minutes, then reduce the oven temperature to 375ºF (190ºC). Add the onions, potatoes, and tomatoes to the bake pan, toss them in the fat in the pan, adding a little more oil if it's needed to moisten them, then season and bake for a final 45 minutes, adding the wine after 20 minutes. The lamb will be pink. If you prefer it more well done, cook it for a little longer.
5. Remove the lamb to a plate, cover with foil, insulate well (I use old towels or tea towels), and leave to rest for 15 minutes. If the potatoes are tender, cover them and keep warm in a low oven while the lamb rests; if they're still a bit firm, increase the oven temperature to 400ºF (205ºC), return the vegetables to the oven, uncovered, and cook until they're ready.
6. Serve the lamb with the potatoes, tomatoes, and onions, scattered with a few basil leaves, if you like.

Sherry Lamb Leg and Autumn Vegetable

Prep time: 10 minutes | Cook time: 3 hours | Serves 8

8 garlic cloves, plus 1 head of garlic, cloves separated
Sea salt flakes and freshly ground black pepper, to taste
Large pinch of saffron threads (optional)
Leaves from 8 thyme sprigs, plus 4 whole thyme sprigs
½ cup extra-virgin olive oil
4½ pounds (2 kg) leg of lamb
1 large onion, cut into wedges
$^{2}/_{3}$ pound (302.4) thin bunched carrots, or, if you can only find thick ones, halve or quarter them lengthwise
1 pound (454 g) waxy potatoes, scrubbed and sliced (no need to peel)
1¾ cups amontillado sherry, plus more if needed

1. Preheat the oven to 450ºF (235ºC).
2. Crush the 8 cloves of garlic in a mortar and pestle with some sea salt flakes (the salt flakes act as an abrasive). Grind in the saffron, if using; it will add its flavor, and of course its gorgeous color, but the dish is just as delicious without. Add the thyme leaves, pepper, and olive oil, to make a loose paste.
3. Make incisions all over the lamb with a knife and slightly loosen the meat around the bone end, too. Push the garlic and herb paste down into these incisions, into the space around the bone and all over the roast. Put into a large bake pan or a cast-iron casserole dish; you will need to add all the vegetables later, too, so there has to be room for them as well. Season all over.
4. Bake for 20 minutes, then remove the pan or casserole from the oven. Reduce the oven temperature to 350ºF (180ºC). Put the onion, carrots, the rest of the garlic cloves, potatoes, and thyme sprigs under and around the lamb. Bring the sherry to just under a boil, then pour it over. Cover tightly

with a double layer of foil, or the lid, and return to the oven.

5. Cook for 2½ hours, turning the lamb over about 3 times and checking on the sherry, too. Most of it will be absorbed during cooking, but don't let it get dry. If there are a lot of juices, remove the foil or uncover the pot 45 minutes before the end of cooking time, so they can reduce. The lamb should be cooked to softness , if it isn't, cook it for a little longer, and the vegetables completely tender. Serve the lamb with the vegetables and the sherry juices.

Lamb Leg with Herb Yogurt Sauce

Prep time: 20 minutes | Cook time: 30 minutes | Serves 8

For the Lamb:

1½ tablespoons cumin seeds
2 teaspoons coriander seeds
1 onion, chopped
Finely grated zest and juice of 1 lime, plus lime wedges to serve
$^{2}/_{3}$ cup plain yogurt
Leaves from 8 mint sprigs, plus mint leaves to serve
Scant 2 cups cilantro leaves and stalks, plus cilantro leaves to serve
6 garlic cloves, chopped
1 red Fresno chili, seeded if you want, chopped
1-inch fresh ginger, peeled and chopped
½ teaspoon sea salt flakes
½ teaspoon freshly ground black pepper
5 pounds (2.3 kg) of lamb (pre-boned weight), boned and butterflied by your butcher

For the Sauce:

1 cup Greek yogurt
Leaves from 8 mint sprigs
2 cups cilantro leaves
5 tablespoons extra-virgin olive oil
2 garlic cloves, chopped
1 scallion, trimmed and chopped
Finely grated zest of 1 lime
2 tablespoons lime juice
3 tablespoons mayonnaise
Sea salt flakes and freshly ground black pepper, to taste

1. Toast the cumin and coriander seeds in a dry frying pan over medium heat for about 2 minutes. Let them cool, then put them in a food processor with the onion, lime zest and juice, yogurt, mint and cilantro, garlic, chili, and ginger, salt and pepper. Whizz until you have a paste.
2. Put the lamb in a dish, or a large plastic food storage bag, with the marinade, making sure the marinade covers the flesh as well as the fatty side. Cover with plastic wrap, or seal the bag, then refrigerate for about 6 hours. Bring the meat to room temperature.
3. Preheat the oven to 425ºF (220ºC).
4. Lift the lamb out of the marinade, shaking it off. Spread the meat out in a bake pan, fatty side up, then bake for 15 minutes.
5. Reduce the oven temperature to 375ºF (190ºC) and cook for another 15 minutes. The lamb will be pink. (If you want it more well done, increase the cooking time by 5 minutes.)
6. Remove from the oven, cover with foil, insulate with kitchen towels or old towels, and leave to rest for 15 minutes.
7. To make the sauce, just put all the ingredients into a clean food processor bowl and blend. Taste for seasoning.
8. Slice the meat and arrange it on a warmed platter, spooning over any juices that have come out of it, and scatter with mint and cilantro leaves and some sea salt flakes. Serve immediately, with lime wedges and the yogurt sauce.

Lamb Shoulder with Lemony Caper Relish

Prep time: 20 minutes | Cook time: 3½ hours | Serves 6

For the Lamb:

2 tablespoons lemon thyme leaves, plus another dozen whole sprigs
6 rosemary sprigs, leaves removed and chopped, plus another dozen whole sprigs
1 tablespoon dried oregano
1 tablespoon sea salt flakes
Freshly ground black pepper, to taste
2 tablespoons extra-virgin olive oil
4½ pounds (2 kg) lamb shoulder on the bone

1 head of garlic, cloves separated
Juice of 1 lemon
1 cup dry white wine
2 tablespoons honey (a floral or herbal type, such as lavender or thyme)
For the Relish:
2 unwaxed lemons
¼ cup extra-virgin olive oil
2 tablespoons honey
1 tablespoon white balsamic vinegar
2 tablespoons lemon juice, or to taste
2 tablespoons capers, drained, rinsed, and patted dry
½ small garlic clove, finely grated
Leaves from 12 mint sprigs, torn

1. Preheat the oven to 400ºF (205ºC). Put all the herb leaves (not the whole sprigs,) and the dried oregano in a mortar with the salt, pepper, and olive oil and grind everything together. Score the lamb fat without cutting into the meat, and rub the herb mixture all over it, pushing it down into the slashes. Scatter the herb sprigs and all the garlic cloves in a bake pan that will hold the lamb snugly. Set the lamb on top; the garlic and the herbs must be underneath, or they will burn. Squeeze the lemon juice over, then pour half the wine into the pan. Cover with a double layer of foil, sealing it tightly around the edges.
2. Put the pan into the oven and immediately reduce the temperature to 300ºF (150ºC), and cook for 3½ to 4 hours. Check every so often to see whether you need to add any more wine (just enough to keep the pan moist). The meat is ready when it is falling off the bone. When there are just 30 minutes cooking time left, drizzle the honey on top. Once it's cooked, lay some towels over the foil and leave the lamb to rest for 15 minutes.
3. To make the relish, remove the lemon zest from 1 lemon with a zester, then roughly chop the zest. Peel the white pith away from the same lemon, then remove all the peel and pith from the other. Remove the flesh from both: using a very sharp knife, cut between each segment and carefully ease it out. Chop the flesh into little pieces and put it in a bowl with the zest, olive oil, honey, vinegar, and lemon juice. Add the capers to the bowl with the garlic. Stir and taste for balance: remember this will be served with fatty lamb that can take a relish that's assertive and quite acidic. Just when you are about to serve, add the mint leaves (they turn black if they sit in acid for too long).

Flank Steak and Bell Pepper Fajitas

Prep time: 15 minutes | Cook time: 30 minutes | Serves 4 to 6

1 tablespoon chili powder
1½ teaspoons sweet paprika
½ teaspoon onion powder
¼ teaspoon garlic powder
¼ teaspoon ground cumin
⅛ teaspoon cayenne pepper
1 teaspoon sugar
½ teaspoon kosher salt
1 large red onion, sliced
2 bell peppers, any color, stemmed, seeded, and cut into strips
1 pound (454 g) flank steak, cut into thin strips
2 tablespoons vegetable oil
Juice of 1 lime
2 tablespoons chopped fresh cilantro
8 flour tortillas, warmed

1. Select Bake and preheat the oven to 400ºF (205ºC).
2. In a small bowl, stir together the chili powder, paprika, onion powder, garlic powder, cumin, cayenne, sugar, and salt.
3. Arrange the red onion, bell peppers, and steak in a single layer on a baking sheet (or use two baking sheets if needed). Drizzle the vegetable oil over everything and toss to coat well.
4. Sprinkle the spice mixture over the top and toss again to distribute. Spread the meat and vegetables into a single layer again. Bake for 30 to 35 minutes, until the peppers and onion are tender and browned and the meat is sizzling. Transfer the meat and vegetables to a serving platter and squeeze the lime juice over the top. Garnish with the cilantro and serve with the tortillas and any desired toppings.

Steak with Brandy Peppercorn Sauce

Prep time: 10 minutes | Cook time: 20 minutes | Serves 4

2 pounds (907 g) steak, such as top loin, strip, or rib eye, about ½ to 1 inch thick
Kosher salt, to taste
Freshly ground black pepper, to taste
3 tablespoons olive oil
3 garlic cloves, skin on and smashed
1 medium shallot, finely chopped
¼ cup brandy
1 cup beef broth
3 tablespoons cracked peppercorns
¼ cup heavy (whipping) cream
¼ cup chopped fresh flat-leaf parsley

1. Select Convection Broil and preheat the oven to 500ºF (260ºC).
2. Place the oven rack in the second-from-the-top position.
3. Season the steak with salt and pepper and place it on a two-piece broiler pan. Place the pan on the positioned oven rack and broil for 5 minutes. Turn the steak and cook for about 3 minutes more for medium (reduce the time slightly for medium-rare or increase the time slightly for medium-well).
4. Remove the steak from the oven, tent loosely with aluminum foil, and let rest for about 10 minutes.
5. While the steak rests, in a medium heavy-bottomed skillet or cast-iron pan over medium heat, heat the olive oil.
6. Add the garlic and shallot. Cook for 2 minutes, stirring.
7. Stir in the brandy and cook for 2 to 3 minutes, stirring and scraping up any browned bits from the bottom of the pan.
8. Add the beef broth and peppercorns. Continue to cook for 5 to 7 minutes, stirring, until the sauce is reduced by about half.
9. Stir in the heavy cream. Continue to cook for about 2 minutes more, stirring, until the sauce is thick. Stir in the parsley. Serve the steak with the sauce spooned over the top.

Juicy Bacon and Beef Cheeseburgers

Prep time: 10 minutes | Cook time: 15 minutes | Serves 4

1½ pounds (680.4 g) ground beef
1 tablespoon Worcestershire sauce
1 teaspoon kosher salt
½ teaspoon freshly ground black pepper
½ teaspoon garlic powder
¾ cup grated sharp Cheddar cheese
4 bacon slices, halved crosswise so you have 8 short strips
4 hamburger buns
Burger fixings as desired: sliced tomatoes, pickles, onions, ketchup, mustard, relish, mayonnaise, etc., for serving

1. Select Bake and preheat the oven to 450ºF (235ºC).
2. Line a baking sheet with aluminum foil and place a wire rack on top.
3. In a medium bowl, mix together the ground beef, Worcestershire sauce, salt, pepper, and garlic powder. Shape the mixture into 8 very thin patties. Top 4 patties with Cheddar, dividing the cheese equally, and top each with 1 of the remaining 4 patties. Press the patties together, sealing the cheese inside. The patties should be equal sizes, about ½ inch thick and 4 to 5 inches across. Place the patties on the wire rack on top of the baking sheet.
4. Arrange the bacon slices on the rack around the patties. Bake the burgers and bacon together for 10 to 15 minutes, until the burgers are cooked through and the bacon is browned and crisp.
5. Remove the patties immediately and place them on the buns.
6. Pat the bacon strips with a paper towel to remove excess fat and lay 2 pieces on top of each burger. Garnish as desired and serve immediately.

Beef Meatloaf with Roasted Vegetables

Prep time: 15 minutes | Cook time: 40 minutes | Serves 4

1½ pounds (680.4 g) ground beef
¼ cup finely diced onion
1 large egg, lightly beaten
½ cup dried bread crumbs, or panko bread crumbs
2 tablespoons tomato paste
2 tablespoons Worcestershire sauce
1½ teaspoons kosher salt, divided
1 teaspoon freshly ground black pepper, divided

2 cups small Brussels sprouts, halved
1 large red onion, halved and sliced
2 cups small new potatoes, halved or quartered
2 tablespoons olive oil

1. Select Convection Bake and preheat the oven to 350ºF (180ºC).
2. Line one or two rimmed baking sheets with aluminum foil or parchment paper.
3. In a medium bowl, mix together the ground beef, onion, egg, bread crumbs, tomato paste, Worcestershire sauce, 1 teaspoon of salt, and ½ teaspoon of pepper until well combined. Form the mixture into a loaf on the prepared sheet.
4. In a large bowl, toss together the Brussels sprouts, red onion, potatoes, olive oil, and the remaining ½ teaspoon of salt and ½ teaspoon of pepper. Arrange the vegetables either around the meatloaf or on a separate baking sheet.
5. Bake for 40 to 45 minutes, until the vegetables are tender and browned and the meat is cooked through. Remove from the oven, tent the meatloaf loosely with foil, and let stand for 10 minutes before serving.

Beef Rump with Red Wine Gravy

Prep time: 15 minutes | Cook time:minutes | Serves 6 to 8

For the Roast:

1 (3- to 3½-pound / 1.4- to 1.6-kg) boneless rump roast, at room temperature
1 tablespoon olive oil
4 garlic cloves, peeled and halved
1½ tablespoons Italian seasoning
1 teaspoon kosher salt
1 teaspoon freshly ground black pepper

For the Red Wine Gravy:

2 tablespoons unsalted butter
3 tablespoons all-purpose flour
¾ cup beef broth
½ cup red wine
Kosher salt, to taste
Freshly ground black pepper, to taste

Make the Roast

1. Select Bake and preheat the oven to 350ºF (180ºC).
2. Brush the roast all over with the olive oil. With the tip of a sharp knife, cut eight slits into the roast and insert a garlic clove half into each slit. Sprinkle the Italian seasoning, salt, and pepper all over the roast and place the roast directly on the oven rack, fat-side up, and place a rimmed baking sheet directly underneath it on the lower rack to catch the drippings. Bake for about 20 minutes, until the outside of the meat is browned.
3. Lower the oven temperature to 200°F and bake for 1 hour, 30 minutes more, until the internal temperature is 135ºF (57ºC) to 140ºF (60ºC). Remove the roast from the oven, tent loosely with aluminum foil, and let rest for 10 minutes.

Make the Red Wine Gravy

4. While the roast rests, carefully remove the pan with the drippings from the oven and reserve.
5. In a medium saucepan over medium-high heat, melt the butter.
6. Add the flour and cook for 3 to 5 minutes, whisking constantly, until the mixture turns golden brown and becomes thick and smooth.
7. Add the pan drippings, beef broth, and red wine. Cook over medium-high heat for 8 to 10 minutes, stirring frequently, until the sauce thickens to the desired consistency. Carve the roast thinly and serve with the gravy.

Rump Roast with Bell Peppers

Prep time: 10 minutes | Cook time: 40 minutes | Serves 6 to 8

2 red bell peppers, stemmed, seeded, and cut into 1-inch-wide strips
2 yellow bell peppers, stemmed, seeded, and cut into 1-inch-wide strips
2 green bell peppers, stemmed, seeded, and cut into 1-inch-wide strips
6 garlic cloves, peeled and left whole
4 tablespoons olive oil, divided
2 teaspoons kosher salt, divided
1½ teaspoons freshly ground black pepper, divided
1 (3- to 3½-pound / 1.4- to 1.6-kg) boneless rump roast, at room temperature
1 tablespoon chopped fresh thyme leaves

1. Select Bake and preheat the oven to 375ºF (190ºC).

2. In a 9-by-13-inch baking dish or on a rimmed baking sheet, toss together the red, yellow, and green bell peppers, garlic, 2 tablespoons of olive oil, ½ teaspoon of salt, and ½ teaspoon of pepper. Spread the peppers out to the sides of the pan, leaving space in the middle for the roast.
3. Rub the remaining 2 tablespoons of olive oil all over the roast and season it with the remaining 1½ teaspoons of salt and 1 teaspoon of pepper. Bake for 40 to 45 minutes, until the outside of the roast is browned and it is cooked to an internal temperature of 135ºF (57ºC).
4. Remove the roast from the oven, tent loosely with aluminum foil, and let rest for 10 minutes. Carve the roast thinly and serve hot, with the roasted peppers and garlic alongside, garnished with the thyme.

Mint-Roasted Boneless Lamb Leg

Prep time: 10 minutes | Cook time: 30 minutes | Serves 8

2 tablespoons olive oil
6 garlic cloves, minced
¼ cup chopped fresh mint leaves
1 tablespoon chopped fresh flat-leaf parsley leaves
1 teaspoon kosher salt
¾ teaspoon freshly ground black pepper
1 (3- to 3½-pound / 1.4- to 1.6-kg) boneless leg of lamb, at room temperature

1. Select Bake and preheat the oven to 400ºF (205ºC).
2. In a small bowl, stir together the olive oil, garlic, mint, parsley, salt, and pepper. Rub the herb mixture all over the meat. Place the meat in a shallow bake pan and bake for 30 to 35 minutes, or until the meat reaches the desired internal temperature to 130ºF (54ºC) for medium-rare, 140ºF (60ºC) for medium, and 145ºF (63ºC) for medium-well.
3. Remove the roast from the oven, tent with aluminum foil, and let rest for at least 15 minutes.
4. To serve, carve the meat thinly across the grain and serve with the pan juices drizzled over the top.

Pork Chops with Lime Peach Salsa

Prep time: 15 minutes | Cook time: 22 minutes | Serves 4

For the Pork Chops:

3 tablespoons low-sodium soy sauce
2 tablespoons ketchup
2 tablespoons light brown sugar
1 tablespoon olive oil
1 garlic clove, minced
1 teaspoon red wine vinegar, or white wine vinegar
4 (7-ounce / 198-g) bone-in pork chops

For the Salsa:

½ medium red bell pepper, seeded and diced
1 to 2 red or green jalapeño peppers, or serrano peppers, diced
2 garlic cloves, minced
4 medium peaches, peeled, pitted, and diced
¼ cup freshly squeezed lime juice
½ teaspoon kosher salt
Fresh cilantro leaves, for garnish

Make the Pork Chops

1. Select Bake and preheat the oven to 400ºF (205ºC).
2. Place an oven rack in the top position and one in the middle or second-from-the-bottom position.
3. In a small bowl, stir together the soy sauce, ketchup, brown sugar, olive oil, garlic, and vinegar. Rub the mixture all over the pork chops, reserving any excess mixture for later.
4. Arrange the chops on a rimmed baking sheet in a single layer. Bake on the lower rack for 10 minutes.
5. Spoon the reserved rub mixture over the top and bake for 10 minutes more.
6. Remove the pan from the oven, select Convection Broil, and increase the oven temperature to 500ºF (260ºC).
7. Place the chops on the upper rack and broil for 2 to 3 minutes, until the tops are golden brown. Serve immediately, topped with a spoonful of the salsa and garnished with cilantro.

Make the Salsa

8. While the pork chops roast, combine the red bell pepper, jalapeño, garlic, and peaches in a medium bowl. Toss to combine.
9. Add the lime juice and salt and toss to coat the mixture well.

Rosemary-Balsamic Pork Loin Roast

Prep time: 10 minutes | Cook time: 35 minutes | Serves 4

¼ cup olive oil
3 tablespoons balsamic vinegar
5 garlic cloves, minced
½ cup chopped fresh rosemary leaves
1 teaspoon kosher salt
½ teaspoon freshly ground black pepper
1 (2-pound / 907-g) boneless pork loin roast

1. Select Bake and preheat the oven to 425ºF (220ºC).
2. In a small bowl, stir together the olive oil, vinegar, garlic, rosemary, salt, and pepper. Rub the mixture all over the pork loin and place it in a 9-by-13-inch baking dish. Bake for 15 minutes.
3. Lower the oven temperature to 350ºF (180ºC) and continue to roast the pork for 20 to 30 minutes more, until the internal temperature is around 145ºF (63ºC). Remove from the oven, tent loosely with aluminum foil, and let rest for 10 minutes before slicing and serving.

Cider-Bourbon Glazed Pork Loin Roast

Prep time: 10 minutes | Cook time: 1¼ hours | Serves 6

3 tablespoons olive oil, divided
1 onion, finely diced
Kosher salt, to taste
1 Granny Smith apple, peeled and finely diced
2 tablespoons chopped fresh sage leaves
Freshly ground black pepper, to taste
1 (2-pound / 907-g) boneless pork loin roast, butterflied and pounded to an even 1-inch thickness
3 tablespoons olive oil
½ cup bourbon
2 cups apple cider
1 tablespoon dark brown sugar

1. Select Bake and preheat the oven to 375ºF (190ºC).
2. In a large skillet over medium-high heat, heat 2 tablespoons of olive oil.
3. Add the onion and a pinch of salt. Cook for 3 minutes, stirring.
4. Add the apple and continue to cook for 3 minutes more, stirring.
5. Stir in the sage and remove from the heat. Taste and season with salt and pepper, if needed.
6. Season the pork loin generously with salt and pepper. Brush the remaining 1 tablespoon of olive oil all over the outside of the roast.
7. Spoon the apple mixture over the pork loin, covering the pork in an even layer. Gently roll the meat around the stuffing and secure with toothpicks or kitchen twine and place in a baking dish.
8. Return the skillet to medium heat and carefully add the bourbon and apple cider. Cook for 2 minutes, stirring and scraping up any browned bits from the bottom of the pan. Pour ¼ cup of the bourbon mixture over the pork.
9. Roast the pork for 1 hour, pouring another ¼ cup of the bourbon mixture over the pork every 20 minutes.
10. After basting with the glaze for a third time, whisk the brown sugar into the bourbon mixture until it dissolves.
11. When the pork is done, transfer it to a cutting board, tent loosely with aluminum foil, and let rest for at least 10 minutes. To serve, cut into 1-inch-thick slices and spoon the sweetened glaze over the top.

Hoisin Roasted Pork Ribs

Prep time: 10 minutes | Cook time: 1 hour | Serves 4 to 6

2 pounds (907 g) baby back pork ribs
1/3 cup hoisin sauce
2 tablespoons soy sauce
2 tablespoons light brown sugar
1 tablespoon minced peeled fresh ginger
2 garlic cloves, minced
1 tablespoon toasted sesame oil
¼ teaspoon ground cinnamon
¼ teaspoon ground fennel

¼ teaspoon cayenne pepper
¼ teaspoon freshly ground black pepper
1. Select Bake and preheat the oven to 350ºF (180ºC).
2. Place the ribs in a large bake pan. Pierce the meat with a fork.
3. In a small bowl, whisk the hoisin sauce, soy sauce, brown sugar, ginger, garlic, sesame oil, cinnamon, fennel, cayenne, and pepper. Brush the mixture over the meat. Reserve any extra marinade for basting. Bake the ribs, uncovered, for 1 hour, basting with the reserved seasoning mixture every 20 minutes.
4. Cut between the bones to separate the ribs and serve immediately.

Brown Sugar-Mustard Glazed Ham

Prep time: 5 minutes | Cook time: 1½ hour | Serves 14 to 16

1 (10- to 12-pound / 4.5- to 5.4-kg) bone-in spiral-sliced ham
1 cup brown sugar
2 tablespoons honey
2 tablespoons Dijon mustard
2 tablespoons apple cider vinegar
1. Select Bake and preheat the oven to 325ºF (163ºC).
2. Place the ham in a shallow bake pan and bake for about 1 hour.
3. In a small bowl, stir together the brown sugar, honey, mustard, and vinegar. After 1 hour, spoon the brown sugar mixture all over the ham. Return the ham to the oven and bake for 20 to 30 minutes more, until heated through and the glaze is bubbling and browned.

Pork Chops with Pickapeppa Sauce

Prep time: 10 minutes | Cook time: 16 minutes | Serves 2

½ to ¾ pound (227- to 340-g) boneless lean pork sirloin chops
Seasoning Mixture:
½ teaspoon ground cumin
¼ teaspoon turmeric
Pinch of ground cardamom
Pinch of grated nutmeg
1 teaspoon vegetable oil
1 teaspoon Pickapeppa sauce
1. Combine the seasoning mixture ingredients in a small bowl and brush on both sides of the chops. Place the chops on the broiling rack with a pan underneath.
2. Broil 8 minutes, remove the chops, turn, and brush with the mixture. Broil again for 8 minutes, or until the chops are done to your preference.

Spicy Pepper Steak

Prep time: 10 minutes | Cook time: 12 minutes | Serves 2

½ to ¾ pound (227- to 340-g) pepper steaks, cut into 3 × 4-inch strips
Spicy Mixture:
1 tablespoon olive oil
1 tablespoon brown mustard
1 teaspoon chili powder
1 teaspoon garlic powder
1 teaspoon hot sauce
1 tablespoon barbecue sauce or salsa
Salt and freshly ground black pepper, to taste
1. Blend the spicy mixture ingredients in a small bowl and brush both sides of the beef strips.
2. Roll up the strips lengthwise and fasten with toothpicks near each end. Place the beef rolls in an oiled or nonstick 8½ × 8½ × 2-inch square baking (cake) pan.
3. Broil for 6 minutes, remove from the oven, and turn with tongs. Brush with the spicy mixture and broil again for 6 minutes, or until done to your preference.

Minted-Balsamic Lamb Chops

Prep time: 5 minutes | Cook time: 15 minutes | Serves 4

4 lean lamb chops, fat trimmed, approximately ¾ inch thick
1 tablespoon balsamic vinegar
Mint Mixture:
4 tablespoons finely chopped fresh mint
2 tablespoons nonfat yogurt

1 tablespoon olive oil
Salt and freshly ground black pepper, to taste

1. Combine the mint mixture ingredients in a small bowl, stirring well to blend. Set aside. Place the lamp chops on a broiling rack with a pan underneath.
2. Broil the lamb chops for 10 minutes, or until they are slightly pink. Remove from the oven and brush one side liberally with balsamic vinegar. Turn the chops over with tongs and spread with the mint mixture, using all of the mixture.
3. Broil again for 5 minutes, or until lightly browned.

Bourbon Sirloin Steak

Prep time: 5 minutes | Cook time: 14 minutes | Serves 2

2 (6- to 8-ounce / 170- to 227-g) sirloin steaks, ¾ inch thick

Brushing Mixture:

¼ cup bourbon
1 teaspoon garlic powder
1 tablespoon olive oil
1 teaspoon soy sauce

1. Combine the brushing mixture ingredients in a small bowl. Brush the steaks on both sides with the mixture and place on the broiling rack with a pan underneath.
2. Broil 4 minutes, remove from the oven, turn with tongs, brush the top and sides, and broil again for 4 minutes, or until done to your preference. To use the brushing mixture as a sauce or gravy, pour the mixture into a baking pan.
3. Broil the mixture for 6 minutes, or until it begins to bubble.

CHAPTER 4 FISH AND SEAFOOD

Lime Jalapeño Crab Cakes with Aioli

Prep time: 15 minutes | Cook time: 18 minutes | Serves 4

For the Crab Cakes:

2 scallions, white and green parts, thinly sliced
1 jalapeño pepper, finely diced
¼ cup mayonnaise
½ teaspoon grated lime zest
1 tablespoon freshly squeezed lime juice
¼ teaspoon kosher salt
¼ teaspoon freshly ground black pepper
1 large egg, lightly beaten
1/3 cup panko bread crumbs
1 pound (454 g) lump crab meat, drained and picked over to remove any bits of shell
2 tablespoons unsalted butter, melted

For the Aioli:

½ cup mayonnaise
2 tablespoons minced fresh cilantro leaves
2 garlic cloves, minced
1 teaspoon freshly squeezed lime juice
⅛ teaspoon kosher salt

Make the Crab Cakes

1. In a medium bowl, stir together the scallions, jalapeño, mayonnaise, lime zest and juice, salt, and pepper.
2. Add the egg and bread crumbs. Stir to combine.
3. Add the crab meat and toss to combine. Cover and refrigerate for 30 minutes.
4. Select Bake and preheat the oven to 400ºF (205ºC).
5. Line a baking sheet with parchment paper.
6. Using wet hands, form the crab mixture into 8 patties, about 1 inch thick, and arrange them on the prepared sheet. Brush the melted butter over the tops of the patties. Bake for 18 to 20 minutes, until golden brown and crisp on the edges. Serve the crab cakes hot, with a dollop of aioli on each.

Make the Aioli

7. While the crab cakes bake, in a small bowl, stir together the mayonnaise, cilantro, garlic, lime juice, and salt.

Panko-Whitefish and Potato

Prep time: 10 minutes | Cook time: 35 minutes | Serves 4

Nonstick cooking spray, for preparing the baking sheet and rack
¼ cup low-fat buttermilk
1½ teaspoons kosher salt, divided
1 pound (454 g) meaty whitefish fillets, such as cod, halibut, or pollock, cut into 2-by-4-inch strips
2 large baking potatoes, peeled and cut into wedges
1 tablespoon olive oil
1 garlic clove, minced
¼ cup all-purpose flour
2 large egg whites
1 cup panko bread crumbs

1. Select Convection Bake and preheat the oven to 400ºF (205ºC).
2. Line a rimmed baking sheet with aluminum foil and spray it with cooking spray. Spray a wire rack (that fits on top of the baking sheet) with cooking spray, and set the rack aside.
3. In a medium bowl, stir together the buttermilk and ½ teaspoon of salt. Add the fish pieces and stir to coat. Cover and refrigerate for about 20 minutes, while you prepare the potatoes and batter.
4. In a large bowl, toss the potato wedges with the olive oil, garlic, and remaining 1 teaspoon of salt. Spread the wedges in a single layer on the prepared sheet. Bake for 20 minutes. Remove from the oven (leave the oven on) and place the prepared rack on top of the baking sheet with the potatoes.
5. While the potatoes roast, put the flour in a shallow dish. In a medium bowl, whisk the egg whites until foamy. Put the bread crumbs in another shallow dish.
6. Working with one piece of fish at a time, remove the fish from the buttermilk, letting the excess drip back into the bowl. Dredge the fish first in the flour, then dip it into the egg white, and finally

coat it with the bread crumbs. Arrange the coated fish pieces in a single layer on the wire rack.

7. Return the baking sheet with the potatoes, along with the rack of fish, to the oven and bake for about 15 minutes more until the fish is golden brown, crisp, and cooked through. Serve hot.

Shrimp with Spicy Orange Sauce

Prep time: 15 minutes | Cook time: 10 minutes | Serves 4

For the Shrimp:

Nonstick cooking spray, for preparing the baking sheet and rack, and the shrimp
2 large egg whites
1½ cups panko bread crumbs
½ teaspoon kosher salt
½ teaspoon freshly ground black pepper
2 pounds (907 g) shrimp, peeled and deveined

For the Spicy Orange Sauce:

Zest of 1 large orange
Juice of 1 large orange
1 (1-inch) piece fresh ginger, peeled and minced
2 tablespoons lower-sodium soy sauce
1 tablespoon honey
⅛ teaspoon cayenne pepper (optional)
1 teaspoon cornstarch mixed with 2 teaspoons cold water

1. Select Bake and preheat the oven to 400ºF (205ºC).

2. Place a wire rack on top of a baking sheet and spray both with cooking spray.

Make the Shrimp

3. In a shallow bowl, lightly beat the egg whites. In another shallow bowl, combine the bread crumbs, salt, and pepper. Dip each shrimp first in the egg whites and then in the seasoned bread crumbs, coating well. Arrange the coated shrimp on the prepared rack in a single layer. Spray them lightly with cooking spray and sprinkle more of the bread crumb mixture on top of the shrimp.

4. Bake for 10 to 12 minutes, until the shrimp are golden brown and crisp on the outside. Serve hot with the sauce drizzled over the top or on the side for dipping.

Make the Spicy Orange Sauce

5. While the shrimp cook, in a small saucepan over medium heat, stir together the orange zest and juice, ginger, soy sauce, honey, and cayenne (if using). Bring to a simmer and cook, stirring, until well combined.

6. Add the cornstarch slurry and cook for about 1 minute more, stirring, until the sauce is thick and syrupy.

Salmon and Mushroom Phyllo Crust

Prep time: 20 minutes | Cook time: 28 minutes | Serves 6

Nonstick cooking spray, for preparing the baking dish
2 tablespoons olive oil
8 ounces (227 g) cremini mushrooms, sliced
1 onion, diced
2 garlic cloves, chopped
1 celery stalk, diced
1 carrot, diced
½ teaspoon kosher salt
½ teaspoon freshly ground black pepper
1 pound (454 g) baby potatoes, diced
2 cups chicken broth
2 cups half-and-half
3 tablespoons all-purpose flour, plus more for the work surface
1 pound (454 g) salmon fillets, cut into bite-size pieces
6 frozen phyllo sheets, thawed according to the package directions
4 tablespoons unsalted butter, melted
½ cup freshly grated Parmesan cheese
2 tablespoons chopped fresh chives

1. Select Convection Bake and preheat the oven to 375ºF (190ºC).

2. Spray a 2½-quart baking dish with cooking spray and place the baking dish on a baking sheet.

3. In a large skillet over medium-high heat, heat the olive oil.

4. Add the mushrooms, onion, garlic, celery, carrot, salt, and pepper. Cook for about 8 minutes, stirring frequently, until the mushrooms begin to brown and the onion is soft.

5. Stir in the potatoes and chicken broth and bring to a boil. Reduce the heat to medium-low, cover, and simmer for about 7 minutes, until the potatoes are tender.
6. In a medium bowl, whisk the half-and-half and flour. Add this mixture to the skillet and cook for about 3 minutes, stirring continuously, until the mixture boils and thickens a bit.
7. Stir in the salmon. Simmer for about 2 minutes, stirring, until the fish is cooked through. Transfer the mixture to the prepared baking dish and spread it into an even layer.
8. On a lightly floured work surface, lay out 1 phyllo sheet and brush it with melted butter. Sprinkle the buttered sheet with 1 heaping tablespoon of Parmesan. Repeat with the remaining 5 phyllo sheets, butter, and cheese. Lay the stack of buttered phyllo sheets on top of the salmon mixture in the baking dish. Tuck in the edges.
9. Slide the baking sheet with the baking dish on top into the oven and bake for about 15 minutes, until the pastry crust is golden brown and the filling is bubbling.
10. .Remove from the oven and let cool for 5 minutes before serving. Serve hot, garnished with the chives.

Salmon Fillet and Vegetable Packets

Prep time: 10 minutes | Cook time: 8 minutes | Serves 4

4 teaspoons unsalted butter, at room temperature, divided
4 (6- to 8-ounce / 170- to 227-g) skinless salmon fillets
1 teaspoon kosher salt, divided
Freshly ground black pepper, to taste
1 tablespoon very finely minced shallot or scallion, divided
1 small tomato, seeded and diced, divided
1 cup chopped or sliced Roasted Mushrooms
¾ cup frozen peas, thawed
2 tablespoons chopped fresh parsley

1. Select Bake and preheat the oven to 425ºF (220ºC).
2. Cut four pieces of parchment paper the size of your sheet pan.
3. For each packet, smear 1 teaspoon of butter in the center of the parchment paper, spreading it out enough for the salmon to fit on the buttered portion. Season each side of the salmon generously with salt and several grinds of pepper, and place it on the butter.
4. Sprinkle the shallot and tomato over each salmon fillet. Scatter the mushrooms and peas around the salmon, and sprinkle the parsley over everything.
5. Lift the longer sides of the parchment so the edges meet right above the salmon, like a tent. Fold the edges over several times, leaving some air space over the fish and vegetables. You'll have what looks like a long tube filled with fish and vegetables. Fold the open ends over toward the fish a few times, crimping the folds tightly with your fingers. If necessary, use metal paper clips to secure the folded ends.
6. Set the packets on a sheet pan and bake for 8 to 11 minutes, depending on the thickness of the fish: 8 minutes for a piece less than 1-inch thick, 10 minutes for 1 inch, and 11 minutes for a thicker piece.
7. To serve, carefully transfer the packets to dinner plates and unfold or cut the parchment open. Alternatively, unfold or cut the parchment while the packets are still on the sheet pan, and slide the fish and vegetables onto each plate.

Cod Fillet with Mixed Roasted Vegetables

Prep time: 15 minutes | Cook time: 20 minutes | Serves 4

1 small eggplant, peeled and cut into ½-inch-thick slices
1 small zucchini, cut into ½-inch-thick slices
2 teaspoons kosher salt, divided
1 small onion, chopped
3 garlic cloves, minced
1 small green bell pepper, seeded and cut into ½-inch chunks (about 1 cup)
1 small red bell pepper, cut into ½-inch chunks (about 1 cup)
½ teaspoon dried oregano

¼ teaspoon freshly ground black pepper
2 tablespoons extra-virgin olive oil
1 pint cherry tomatoes, halved
4 (6-ounce / 170-g) cod fillets
$^{1}/_{3}$ cup pesto, plus more for serving (optional)

1. Select Bake and preheat the oven to 375ºF (190ºC).
2. Salt one side of the eggplant and zucchini slices with ¾ teaspoon of salt. Place the slices salted-side down on paper towels. Salt the other sides with another ¾ teaspoon of salt. Let the slices sit for 10 minutes, or until they start to exude water. Rinse and blot dry with more paper towels. Cut the zucchini slices into quarters and the eggplant slices into eighths.
3. Transfer the zucchini and eggplant to a sheet pan and add the onion, garlic, and bell peppers. Drizzle with the oil and sprinkle with the oregano and black pepper, tossing to coat.
4. Bake for 8 minutes. Stir the tomatoes into the vegetable mixture. Place the cod fillets in a single layer on top of the vegetables and sprinkle with the remaining ½ teaspoon of salt. Drizzle the pesto over the fish and vegetables, using a basting brush to spread the pesto evenly over the fillets.
5. Bake for 12 minutes, or until the fish flakes easily with a fork.
6. To serve, spoon the vegetables onto a platter and top with the fish fillets, with additional pesto on the side, if desired.

Snapper Fillet with Celery Salad

Prep time: 10 minutes | Cook time: 15 minutes | Serves 4

4 (6- to 8-ounce / 170- to 227-g) boneless, skinless snapper fillets
1½ teaspoons kosher salt, divided
4 tablespoons extra-virgin olive oil, divided
4 large celery stalks, thinly sliced, divided, leaves reserved and torn
2 garlic cloves, thinly sliced
3 scallions, chopped
$^{1}/_{3}$ cup low-sodium chicken or vegetable broth
¼ cup dry white wine
½ teaspoon celery seed, divided
1 tablespoon freshly squeezed lemon juice

1. Select Bake and preheat the oven to 325ºF (163ºC).
2. Sprinkle both sides of each fillet with ¾ teaspoon of salt and set aside.
3. In a 10-inch cast-iron or other oven-safe skillet, heat 2 tablespoons of oil over medium-high heat until shimmering. Add three-quarters of the sliced celery, the garlic, and scallions. Stir-fry for 2 to 3 minutes, until the celery starts to soften. Pour in the broth and wine and bring to a simmer. Stir in ¼ teaspoon of celery seed and ⅜ teaspoon of the remaining salt.
4. Place the fish fillets in a single layer on top of the celery mixture and transfer the skillet to the oven. Bake for 12 to 16 minutes, until the fish flakes with a fork.
5. Meanwhile, put the remaining celery and the celery leaves in a small bowl. In a small jar with a tight lid, combine the remaining 2 tablespoons of oil, lemon juice, remaining ¼ teaspoon of celery seed, and remaining ⅜ teaspoon of salt and shake to combine.
6. When the fish is done, transfer the fillets and braised celery to a platter.
7. Shake the dressing again and pour it over the raw celery and celery leaves, tossing to coat. Top the fish with the celery salad and serve.

Tuna and Asparagus with Lemon-Caper Sauce

Prep time: 10 minutes | Cook time: 20 minutes | Serves 4

1 pound (454 g) asparagus, trimmed
8 tablespoons olive oil, divided
1 teaspoon kosher salt, divided
1 garlic clove, minced
2 tablespoons freshly squeezed lemon juice
¼ cup chopped fresh parsley, divided
2 tablespoons drained capers
½ teaspoon freshly ground black pepper
4 (8-ounce / 227 g) tuna steaks, about ¾-inch thick

1. Position the top oven rack about 8 inches from the broiling element. Select Bake and preheat the oven to 400ºF (205ºC).

2. Arrange the asparagus on a sheet pan and drizzle with 1 tablespoon of oil. Toss to coat and sprinkle with ½ teaspoon of salt.
3. Bake the asparagus for 7 to 10 minutes depending on thickness, until just barely tender.
4. Meanwhile, in a small saucepan, heat 3 tablespoons of the remaining oil over low heat. Add the garlic and sauté just until fragrant. Stir in the lemon juice, half the parsley, and capers. Remove the pan from the heat and set aside.
5. Remove the sheet pan from the oven and switch the oven to Convection Broil. Select the High setting if possible.
6. Rub the remaining 4 tablespoons of oil over both sides of the tuna steaks, and sprinkle with the remaining ½ teaspoon of salt and the pepper. Place the tuna steaks in a single layer on top of the asparagus. Broil for 8 to 10 minutes, turning the fish carefully about halfway through the cooking time. The tuna steaks should still be pink in the middle, and the asparagus should be tender and browned in spots.
7. To serve, drizzle the warm lemon-caper sauce over the tuna and asparagus, then sprinkle the remaining parsley over the fish.

Clam Appetizers

Prep time: 10 minutes | Cook time: 10 minutes | Makes 12 appetizers

1 (6-ounce / 170-g) can minced clams, well drained
1 cup multigrain bread crumbs
1 tablespoon minced onion
1 teaspoon garlic powder
1 teaspoon Worcestershire sauce
1 tablespoon chopped fresh parsley
2 tablespoons olive oil
Salt and freshly ground black pepper, to taste
Lemon wedges

1. Preheat the toaster oven to 450ºF (235ºC).
2. Combine all the ingredients in a medium bowl and fill 12 scrubbed clamshells or small baking dishes with equal portions of the mixture. Place in an 8½ × 8½ × 2-inch oiled or nonstick square (cake) pan.
3. Bake for 10 minutes, or until lightly browned.

Breaded Crab Cakes

Prep time: 10 minutes | Cook time: 30 minutes | Serves 6

1 pound (454 g) fresh lump crab meat, drained and chopped
1 cup bread crumbs
½ cup plain nonfat yogurt
1 tablespoon olive oil
2 tablespoons capers
1 tablespoon garlic powder
1 teaspoon hot sauce
1 egg, beaten
1 tablespoon Worcestershire sauce
Salt and freshly ground black pepper, to taste

1. Preheat the toaster oven to 350ºF (180ºC).
2. Combine all the ingredients in a bowl. Shape the mixture into patties approximately 2½ inches wide, adding more bread crumbs if the mixture is too wet and sticky and more yogurt if the mixture is too dry and crumbly. Place the patties in an 8½ × 8½ × 2-inch oiled or nonstick square (cake) pan.
3. Bake, uncovered, for 25 minutes.
4. Broil for 5 minutes, until golden brown.

Salmon with Cucumber Sauce

Prep time: 15 minutes | Cook time: 20 minutes | Serves 2

2 (6-ounce / 170-g) salmon steaks
2 tablespoons fresh watercress, rinsed, drained, and chopped (for serving hot)
1 lemon, cut into small wedges (for serving hot)

Poaching Liquid:

1 cup dry white wine
2 bay leaves
1 tablespoon mustard seed
Salt and freshly ground black pepper, to taste

Cucumber Sauce:

1 cucumber, peeled, halved, seeds scooped out with a teaspoon and discarded, and finely chopped
½ teaspoon white vinegar
½ teaspoon honey
¼ teaspoon salt
½ cup plain fat-free yogurt
½ cup fat-free or reduced-fat sour cream

1 tablespoon finely chopped fresh dill or 1 teaspoon dried dill weed

1. Preheat the toaster oven to 350ºF (180ºC).
2. Combine the poaching liquid ingredients with 1 cup water in a small bowl and set aside.
3. Place the salmon steaks in an oiled or nonstick 8½ × 8½ × 2-inch square baking (cake) pan and pour enough poaching liquid over the steaks to barely cover them. Adjust the seasonings to taste.
4. Bake, uncovered, for 20 minutes, or until the fish feels springy to the touch. Remove the bay leaves and serve the fish hot with watercress and lemon or cold with cucumber sauce.

Fish Fillet en Casserole

Prep time: 10 minutes | Cook time: 20 minutes | Serves 4

½ cup multigrain bread crumbs
4 (6-ounce / 170-g) fish fillets

Sauce:

2 tablespoons white wine
1 teaspoon Worcestershire sauce
1 teaspoon lemon juice
1 tablespoon vegetable oil
1 teaspoon Dijon mustard
Salt and freshly ground black pepper, to taste
2 tablespoons capers

1. Preheat the toaster oven to 400ºF (205ºC).
2. Layer the bottom of an oiled or nonstick 8½ × 8½ × 2-inch square baking (cake) pan with the bread crumbs and place the fillets on the crumbs.
3. Combine the sauce ingredients, mixing well, and spoon over the fillets. Sprinkle with the capers.
4. Bake, covered, for 20 minutes, or until the fish flakes easily with a fork.

Tuna and Veggies Macaroni

Prep time: 10 minutes | Cook time:1 hour | Serves 4

1 cup elbow macaroni
2 (6-ounce / 170-g) cans tuna packed in water, drained well and crumbled
1 cup frozen peas
1 (6-ounce / 170-g) can button mushrooms, drained
1 tablespoon margarine
Salt and freshly ground black pepper, to taste
1 cup fat-free half-and-half
4 tablespoons unbleached flour
1 teaspoon garlic powder
1 cup multigrain bread crumbs

1. Preheat the toaster oven to 400ºF (205ºC).
2. Combine the macaroni and 3 cups water in a 1-quart 8½ × 8½ × 4-inch ovenproof baking dish, stirring to blend well. Cover with aluminum foil.
3. Bake, covered, for 35 minutes, or until the macaroni is tender. Remove from the oven and drain well. Return to the baking dish and add the tuna, peas, and mushrooms. Add salt and pepper to taste.
4. Whisk together the half-and-half, flour, and garlic powder in a small bowl until smooth. Add to the macaroni mixture and stir to blend well.
5. Bake, covered, for 25 minutes. Remove from the oven, sprinkle the top with the bread crumbs, and dot with the margarine. Bake, uncovered, for 10 minutes, or until the top is browned.

Salmon and Zucchini Burgers

Prep time: 10 minutes | Cook time: 25 minutes | Serves 4

¾ cup bread crumbs
1 (15-ounce / 425-g) can salmon, drained
1 small zucchini, finely chopped
2 tablespoons finely chopped onions
1 egg
1 teaspoon dried rosemary
1 teaspoon lemon juice
1 teaspoon garlic powder
Salt and freshly ground black pepper, to taste
1 teaspoon vegetable oil

1. Preheat the toaster oven to 400ºF (205ºC).
2. Blend all ingredients except the oil and form patties 1½ inches thick. Place on an oiled or nonstick 8½ × 8½ × 2-inch square baking (cake) pan.
3. Bake for 25 minutes, or until the patties are lightly browned.

Tuna Cheese Picnic Loaf

Prep time: 10 minutes | Cook time: 10 minutes | Serves 4

1 French baguette, sliced in half lengthwise, then quartered

Filling:

1 (6-ounce / 170-g) can tuna in water, well drained
2 tablespoons chopped onion
2 tablespoons chopped Spanish olives with pimientos, drained
2 tablespoons chopped fresh parsley
2 tablespoons chopped bell pepper
1 teaspoon dried tarragon
Salt and butcher's pepper, to taste
½ cup shredded low-fat Mozzarella cheese

1. Remove enough bread from each quarter to make a small cavity for the sandwich filling.
2. Combine all the filling ingredients and spoon the mixture in equal portions into each of the bread quarter cavities. Sprinkle each quarter with equal portions of Mozzarella cheese.
3. Broil on a broiling rack with a pan underneath for 10 minutes, or until the bread is lightly browned and the cheese is melted. If your toaster oven cannot accommodate 4 French bread quarters, broil them in two batches. Slice and serve.

Salmon Fillet with Beans

Prep time: 10 minutes | Cook time: 15 minutes | Serves 4

1 pound (454 g) string beans, stem end removed
4 tablespoons extra-virgin olive oil
Sea salt flakes and freshly ground black pepper, to taste
4 (6- to7-ounce / 170- to 198-g) salmon fillets,
¾ cup breadcrumbs from coarse white bread (such as Ciabatta or sourdough)
1 garlic clove, finely grated
3 tablespoons drained and chopped cornichons
2 teaspoons Dijon mustard
2 tablespoons finely chopped flat-leaf parsley leaves
Finely grated zest and juice of ½ unwaxed lemon

1. Preheat the oven to 400ºF (205ºC).
2. Put the string beans into a bake pan. Toss them with a little of the oil and some seasoning.
3. Brush the salmon fillets with oil as well, season, then set them on top of the beans. Bake for 12 minutes.
4. Heat the remaining oil in a frying pan on the stovetop. When it's hot, add the breadcrumbs and fry briskly until golden, then add the garlic and cornichons and cook for another minute. Take the pan off the heat and stir in the mustard, parsley, and lemon zest, mixing together well.
5. When 2 minutes of cooking time remain, spoon the breadcrumb mixture on top of the salmon and return it to the oven.
6. Squeeze the lemon juice over the top of the fish and serve.

Salmon with Mushroom and Bok Choy

Prep time: 10 minutes | Cook time: 12 minutes | Serves 4

2 tablespoons white miso paste
2 tablespoons clear honey
7 tablespoons mirin, or dry vermouth or dry sherry
1 tablespoon light soy sauce
2 teaspoons peeled and finely grated fresh ginger
2 teaspoons toasted sesame oil
A little peanut oil
½ pound (227 g) shiitake mushrooms, trimmed and thinly sliced
2 heads of bok choy, sliced lengthwise
8 scallions, trimmed and roughly chopped
4¼ pounds (1.9 kg) salmon fillets, (not skinny fillets from the tail)
A few sesame seeds (optional)
Rice or noodles, to serve

1. Preheat the oven to 375ºF (190ºC).
2. Mix together the miso, honey, 2 tablespoons of the rice wine, the soy sauce, ginger, and sesame oil.
3. Put 4 rectangles of foil or parchment paper—each about 13½ x 9½in and of double thickness—on to 1 or 2 baking sheets (depending on the size of the sheets). Brush the center of each piece with peanut oil.
4. Divide the mushrooms and bok choy among the pieces of foil, placing them in the center (it will seem like a lot, but the vegetables really shrink as they cook). Sprinkle with the scallions.
5. Drizzle about 1 tablespoon of the miso mixture over the top of each heap of vegetables, then set a salmon fillet on top. Spread the rest of the miso mixture on top of each piece of fish (use all of it).
6. Pull the foil or paper up around the salmon, enclosing the vegetables and nipping the ends of each parcel, but let the top of each fish fillet remain

exposed. Spoon the remaining rice wine into each parcel, dividing it evenly.

7. Bake for 12 minutes. Sprinkle the salmon with sesame seeds, if you're using them, and serve the fish in the parcels, with rice or noodles on the side.

Cod, Chorizo and Roasted Vegetable

Prep time: 15 minutes | Cook time: 45 minutes | Serves 4

For the Cod and Chorizo:

1 pound (454 g) baby potatoes, scrubbed and quartered

$^{2}/_{3}$ pound (302.4 g) cherry tomatoes on the vine

¼ pound (113.4 g) Spanish chorizo cooking sausages, sliced

Leaves from 3 thyme sprigs, plus 3 whole thyme sprigs

Sea salt flakes and freshly ground black pepper, to taste

3 tablespoons extra-virgin olive oil

4 (6-ounce / 170-g) thick cod fillets (not skinny fillets from the tail)

8 to 10 good-quality whole green olives

$^{1}/_{3}$ cup amontillado sherry lemon wedges, to serve

For the Crust:

$1^{1}/_{3}$ cups fresh white breadcrumbs

2 garlic cloves, crushed

Finely grated zest of 1 small unwaxed lemon

1 tablespoon chopped flat- leaf parsley leaves

Leaves from 2 thyme sprigs

¼ teaspoon smoked paprika

4 tablespoons unsalted butter, melted

½ tablespoon amontillado sherry

1. Preheat the oven to 400ºF (205ºC). Put all the vegetables, the chorizo, and all the thyme into a bake pan in which they can lie in a single layer. Season and add 2 tablespoons of the extra-virgin olive oil (more oil will come out of the chorizo once it starts cooking). Toss everything around with your hands and roast in the oven for 30 minutes, turning the vegetables over a couple of times.

2. Now make the crust. Combine the breadcrumbs, garlic, lemon zest, herbs, and smoked paprika and season well. Pour in the melted butter and sherry and mix with a large fork or your fingers until combined. Brush the cod filets with the last tablespoon of oil, then cover them evenly with the crumbs, pressing down on them so they stick to the fish.

3. Mix the olives and sherry into the roasted vegetables and chorizo, then put the cod on top. Return to the oven and bake until the fish is cooked through: its flakes should be opaque, not translucent. This should take 15 minutes, but check for doneness and return the fish to the oven for no more than a couple of minutes if it needs a little longer. Serve with lemon wedges.

Salmon with Beet and Horseradish Purée

Prep time: 10 minutes | Cook time: 11 minutes | Serves 6

For the Purée:

1 pound (454 g) cooked beets (not pickled)

1 small garlic clove, finely grated

Juice of ½ lemon, or to taste

1 tablespoon white balsamic vinegar, or to taste

1 tablespoon peeled and finely grated fresh horseradish

1 tablespoon crème fraîche

Sea salt flakes and freshly ground black pepper, to taste

For the Fish:

2¼ pounds (1 kg) salmon fillet, pin-bones removed

3 tablespoons unsalted butter

3 tablespoons equal parts chopped flat-leaf parsley and dill leaves, plus dill sprigs to serve

Lemon wedges, to serve

1. Preheat the oven to 450ºF (235ºC).

2. For the purée, put everything except the crème fraîche into a food processor, season, and whizz until smooth. Scrape this into a bowl and add the crème fraîche. Taste for seasoning. You might need to adjust the lemon juice and vinegar, too.

3. Find a heavy bake pan big enough to hold the salmon. Run your hand over the surface of the fish from head to tail to make sure that there are no bones; if there are, remove them with your fingers. Season the fish.

4. Melt the butter in the bake pan over medium-low heat on the stovetop, then add half the herbs and put the salmon on top, skin side up. Transfer to the oven and bake for 5 minutes. Remove from the oven and take the skin off, it should peel off quite easily. Then season the flesh and flip the salmon over. Sprinkle with the remaining herbs and return to the oven for a final 6 to 8 minutes. Carefully slide the point of a sharp knife into the thickest part of the fish: it should be opaque, not translucent.
5. Serve on a warmed platter with dill (or chervil) sprigs and lemon wedges. Offer the beet and horseradish purée on the side.

Mackerel with Mango and Chili Salad

Prep time: 15 minutes | Cook time: 20 minutes | Serves 4

For the Fish:

2 garlic cloves, finely grated
1½in fresh ginger, peeled and finely grated
¾ teaspoon ground turmeric
1½ teaspoons ground cumin
½ teaspoon ground fenugreek
2½ tablespoons tamarind paste
¼ cup lime juice, plus more to serve, plus lime wedges to serve
1 tablespoon light brown sugar
2 tablespoons peanut oil
Sea salt flakes and freshly ground black pepper, to taste
4 whole Boston mackerel, gutted and washed
Rice, or warmed naan bread and plain yogurt, to serve

For the Salad:

2 just-ripe or slightly under- ripe mangoes
Juice of 2 limes
1 red Fresno chilli and 1 green chilli, halved, seeded, and very finely shredded
½ cup cilantro leaves and stalks (make sure the stalks aren't too long or thick)

1. Mix together the garlic, ginger, and all the spices for the mackerel, adding the lime juice, sugar, oil, and seasoning. Spread this all over each fish, inside and out. Cover and put in the refrigerator for about 15 minutes.
2. Preheat the oven to 400ºF (205ºC).
3. Now make the salad. Peel the mangoes and cut off the 'cheeks' (the fleshy bits that lie alongside the stone). Cut the cheeks into neat slices.
4. Put the mango slices in a serving bowl and add the lime juice, chilies, some salt, and the cilantro, and toss.
5. Line a bake pan with foil or parchment paper and put the mackerel in it. Bake the mackerel for 20 minutes (if the fish are very big, they might need a little longer; make sure the flesh near the bone is opaque).
6. Squeeze some lime juice over the fish and serve with rice, or warmed naan bread and yogurt, lime wedges, and the mango and chili salad.

Sea Bass Stuffed with Spice Paste

Prep time: 20 minutes | Cook time: 20 minutes | Serves 6 to 8

For the Spice Paste:

1½-inch fresh ginger, peeled and finely grated
2 garlic cloves, finely grated
Scant ¼ teaspoon cayenne pepper
Juice of ½ small lemon
2 tablespoons extra-virgin olive oil
Sea salt flakes and freshly ground black pepper, to taste

For the Stuffing:

9 tablespoons unsalted butter, softened
Generous ¼ cup almond flour
½ cup raisins, soaked in boiling water for 15 minutes, then Drained and patted dry
2 slices of crystallized ginger, very finely chopped
2 preserved lemons, flesh and rind finely chopped, pips removed
1 garlic clove, finely grated
2 tablespoons chopped cilantro leaves

For the Fish:

2 (2-pound / 57-g) sea bass (branzino), gutted, scaled and washed
A little extra-virgin olive oil
1 unwaxed lemon, finely sliced, plus lemon wedges to serve
Couscous, to serve

1. Preheat the oven to 425ºF (220ºC). Make the spice paste by mixing everything together in a bowl. Make the stuffing in the same way in a separate bowl, adding plenty of seasoning to both mixtures.
2. Wash the fish to get rid of any blood (it's bitter) and pat dry with paper towels. Put a double layer of parchment into a bake pan big enough for the fish. Brush the center—where the fish will lie—with olive oil.
3. Make diagonal slashes in the fish on each side, cutting down to the bone but not through it. Push the spice paste inside the slits on both sides of each fish. Carefully stuff the butter mixture inside, pushing it up into the heads to get all of it in (you're not going to eat the heads, but you will be able to get the stuffing out of it). Put the fish on to the oiled parchment paper. Lay the lemon slices inside and on top, then drizzle with olive oil and season.
4. Bake for 20 minutes, then check for doneness: the flesh near the bone in the thickest part of the fish should be opaque. If it needs a little longer, return it to the oven for no more than a couple of minutes, then check again.
5. Serve with lemon wedges and a bowl of couscous tossed with some chopped pistachios, lemon juice, and finely grated lemon zest.

Monkfish with Roast Lemon Salsa Verde

Prep time: 15 minutes | Cook time: 55 minutes | Serves 6

For the Salsa Verde:

1 unwaxed lemon (not too small), cut into slices ⅛in thick
$^2/_3$ cup extra-virgin olive oil
10 anchovies, drained of oil
15 basil leaves
15 mint leaves
Leaves from a 1 ounce bunch of flat-leaf parsley
¼ tablespoon Dijon mustard
1 garlic clove, chopped
1 tablespoon capers, rinsed, drained, and patted dry

For the Fish:

5 tablespoons extra-virgin olive oil
Sea salt flakes and freshly ground black pepper, to taste
$3^1/_3$ pounds (1.5 kg) monkfish tail on the bone, skinned and membrane removed
3 garlic cloves, finely sliced
Leaves from 4 rosemary sprigs

1. Preheat the oven to 325ºF (163ºC).
2. Put the lemon slices for the salsa verde onto a sheet pan lined with parchment paper. Cook for 25 minutes. Allow to cool a little, then peel the slices off the parchment, put them in a bowl, and cover with the olive oil. Leave to soak for a few hours if you can: the oil slightly softens the rind and, in turn, the slices flavor the oil.
3. When you're ready to cook, preheat the oven to 450ºF (235ºC). Put a heavy bake pan over high heat and add 2 tablespoons of the olive oil. Season the fish and brown it all over, it will take about 5 minutes. Then put it into the oven. Bake for 25 minutes; the flesh near the bone should be white, not translucent.
4. Make the salsa verde by putting all the ingredients, except the oil and lemon slices, in a food processor. Pulse-mix, pouring in the lemon-flavored olive oil as you do so (but not the lemon slices yet). Scrape into a bowl. Chop the roast lemon slices and add them to the mixture, seasoning with a little pepper.
5. Heat the remaining 3 tablespoons of olive oil in a frying pan and sauté the garlic and rosemary until the garlic is golden. Serve the fish, either in the dish in which it has cooked or on a warmed platter, with the garlic and rosemary oil spooned over the top and the roast lemon salsa verde on the side.

Sea Bass with Asian Chili Dressing

Prep time: 15 minutes | Cook time: 20 minutes | Serves 6

For the Fish:

1 red Fresno chili, halved, seeded, and chopped
1¼-inch fresh ginger, peeled and finely grated
3 garlic cloves, finely grated
¾ cup cilantro leaves, roughly chopped, plus ¼ cup Cilantro leaves to serve
Finely grated zest of 2 limes, plus the juice of ½ lime, plus Lime wedges to serve
Sea salt flakes

2 tablespoons peanut oil
2 (2 pounds / 907-g) sea bass (branzino), gutted, scaled and washed
6 scallions, trimmed and roughly chopped

For the Dressing:

Juice of 1 lime
2 tablespoons superfine sugar
$^{1}/_{3}$ cup fish sauce
1 red Fresno chili, halved, seeded, and very thinly sliced

1. Preheat the oven to 400ºF (205ºC).
2. Put a double layer of parchment paper into a bake pan or onto a sheet pan with a lip. It obviously needs to be big enough to hold the fish.
3. Put the chili, ginger, garlic, the ¾ cup of cilantro, and the lime zest into a mortar with some salt and pound them together, adding 1 tablespoon of the oil, until you have a rough paste. Add the lime juice.
4. Put the fish on the parchment paper. Make 4 slits in both sides of each fish, without cutting through the bone, and push the paste into them. Stuff the fish with the scallions. Rub the rest of the oil over the fish on both sides and season with salt. Bake for 20 minutes, then check for doneness: the flesh near the bone at the thickest part should be opaque, not translucent.
5. Make the dressing by mixing together the lime juice, sugar, fish sauce, and chili. Serve the fish with the dressing on the side, or spoon it over the top. Scatter with the ¼ cup cilantro leaves and serve with lime wedges.

Shrimp Fajitas with Avocado and Salsa

Prep time: 10 minutes | Cook time: 10 minutes | Serves 4

8 (6-inch) flour or corn tortillas
1 red bell pepper, cut into ½-inch-thick slices
1 green bell pepper, cut into ½-inch-thick slices
1 jalapeño pepper, seeded and cut into ⅛-inch-thick slices
1 medium onion, cut into ½-inch-thick wedges
3 tablespoons vegetable oil, divided
2 tablespoons Mexican or fajita seasoning, divided
1 teaspoon kosher salt, divided
1½ pounds (680.4 g) large shrimp, peeled and deveined
1 small avocado, sliced, for serving
Salsa, for serving

1. Select Bake and preheat the oven to 375ºF (190ºC).
2. Wrap the tortillas tightly in a large sheet of aluminum foil.
3. Put the bell peppers, jalapeño, and onion on a large sheet pan and drizzle with 2 tablespoons of oil. Sprinkle with 1 tablespoon of Mexican seasoning and ½ teaspoon of salt and toss to coat.
4. Place the sheet pan on the upper rack and the tortillas on the lower rack.
5. Bake for 5 minutes, then remove the sheet pan from the oven. Stir the vegetables and move them to the outer edges of the pan. Place the shrimp in the center of the pan and drizzle with the remaining 1 tablespoon of oil. Sprinkle with the remaining 1 tablespoon of Mexican seasoning and ½ teaspoon of salt. Stir to distribute the seasonings evenly.
6. Continue roasting for 5 to 6 minutes, until the vegetables are soft and browned in places and the shrimp are opaque. Remove the sheet pan and tortillas from the oven.
7. Spoon the fajita mixture into the tortillas. Serve with avocado slices and salsa.

Lemony Shrimp with Arugula

Prep time: 10 minutes | Cook time: 10 minutes | Serves 4

4 tablespoons unsalted butter
2 tablespoons extra-virgin olive oil
1 teaspoon kosher salt
6 garlic cloves, minced
¼ cup chopped fresh parsley, divided
2 pounds (907 g) large shrimp, peeled and deveined
2 tablespoons freshly squeezed lemon juice
1 (9- to 10-ounce / 255- to 283-g) bag arugula

1. Select Bake and preheat the oven to 375ºF (190ºC). Put the butter in a 9-by-13-inch baking pan, and place the pan in the oven while the oven heats.
2. When the butter has melted, remove the pan from the oven and add the oil, salt, garlic, and half the parsley. Stir well. Add the shrimp and toss to coat, then arrange the shrimp in a single layer. Bake

for 5 minutes. Check the shrimp; they should be opaque and pink. If they are not quite done, cook for another minute.

3. Remove the pan from the oven. Add the lemon juice, arugula, and remaining parsley. Toss well to wilt the arugula. Serve immediately.

Bacon-Wrapped Herb Rainbow Trout

Prep time: 10 minutes | Cook time: 20 minutes | Serves 4

4 (8- to 10-ounce / 227- to 283-g) rainbow trout, butterflied and boned
2 teaspoons kosher salt, divided
1 tablespoon extra-virgin olive oil, divided
1 tablespoon freshly squeezed lemon juice, divided
2 tablespoons chopped fresh parsley, divided
2 tablespoons chopped fresh chives, divided
8 thin bacon slices
Lemon wedges, for serving

1. Select Bake and preheat the oven to 400ºF (205ºC). Lightly oil a sheet pan and place it in the oven as it preheats.
2. Sprinkle the inside and outside of each trout with the salt. Brush the inside with the oil and drizzle with the lemon juice. Scatter the parsley and chives on one side of each butterflied trout. Fold the trout closed and wrap each one with two slices of bacon.
3. Remove the pan from the oven and place the trout on it. Bake for 20 to 25 minutes, flipping halfway through, until the bacon is crisp. Serve with lemon wedges.

Crab Cheese Enchiladas

Prep time: 10 minutes | Cook time: 25 minutes | Serves 4

8 (6-inch) corn tortillas
Nonstick cooking spray or vegetable oil, for brushing
2 cups mild tomatillo salsa or green enchilada sauce
½ cup heavy (whipping) cream
8 ounces (227 g) lump crab meat, picked through to remove any shells
3 or 4 scallions, chopped
8 ounces (227 g) Monterey Jack cheese, shredded

1. Select Bake and preheat the oven to 350ºF (180ºC).
2. Spray the tortillas on both sides with cooking spray or brush lightly with oil. Arrange on a sheet pan, overlapping as little as possible. Bake for 5 minutes, or until warm and flexible.
3. Meanwhile, stir together the salsa and cream in a shallow, microwave-safe bowl and heat in the microwave until very warm, about 45 seconds.
4. Pour a quarter of the salsa mixture into a 9-by-13-inch baking dish. Place a tortilla in the sauce, turning it over to coat thoroughly. Spoon a heaping tablespoon of crab down the middle of the tortilla, then top with a teaspoon of scallions and a heaping tablespoon of cheese. Roll up the tortilla and place it seam-side down at one end of the pan. Repeat with the remaining tortillas, forming a row of enchiladas in the pan. Spoon most or all of the remaining sauce over the enchiladas so they are nicely coated but not drowning. Sprinkle the remaining cheese over the top.
5. Bake for 18 to 20 minutes, until the cheese is melted and the sauce is bubbling.

Salmon Fillet with Spinach, and Beans

Prep time: 10 minutes | Cook time: 35 minutes | Serves 4

2 tablespoons olive oil, divided
1 garlic clove, thinly sliced
1 (9- to 10-ounce / 255- to 283-g) bag baby spinach
1 (15-ounce / 425-g) can cannellini or navy beans, rinsed and drained
1½ teaspoons kosher salt, divided
½ teaspoon ground cumin
½ teaspoon ground coriander
¼ teaspoon red pepper flakes
4 (6-ounce / 170-g) skinless salmon fillets

1. Select Bake and preheat the oven to 300ºF (150ºC).
2. Heat 1 tablespoon of oil in a large, oven-safe skillet over medium-high heat. Add the garlic and cook, stirring, until fragrant, about 30 seconds. Add the spinach a handful at a time and cook, tossing, until slightly wilted, adding more as you have room.

Stir in the beans, ¾ teaspoon of salt, cumin, coriander, and red pepper flakes.

3. Season the salmon with the remaining ¾ teaspoon of salt. Place the fillets in a single layer on top of the spinach mixture and drizzle with the remaining 1 tablespoon of oil.

4. Bake until the salmon is opaque in the center, 30 to 35 minutes.

Sherry Tilapia and Mushroom Rice

Prep time: 15 minutes | Cook time: 25 minutes | Serves 4

4 tablespoons unsalted butter
12 ounces (340 g) cremini or white button mushrooms, trimmed and sliced
4 to 6 scallions, chopped
1 teaspoon kosher salt, divided
2 tablespoons all-purpose flour
¾ cup dry sherry or dry white wine
¾ cup low-sodium vegetable or fish broth
3 tablespoons heavy (whipping) cream
1 tablespoon chopped fresh parsley, divided
2 cups cooked white or brown rice
4 (6-ounce / 170-g) tilapia fillets
⅛ teaspoon freshly ground black pepper

1. Select Bake and preheat the oven to 325ºF (163ºC).

2. In a large cast-iron or other oven-safe skillet, melt the butter over medium heat until foaming. Sauté the mushrooms and scallions until the mushrooms are soft. Stir in ½ teaspoon of salt and the flour. Cook for 1 minute, stirring constantly. Gradually stir in the sherry. Let the sauce simmer for 3 to 5 minutes, until some of the alcohol evaporates. Add the broth, cream, and 1½ teaspoons of parsley and bring back to a simmer.

3. Stir the rice into the sauce. Place the fish fillets in a single layer on top of the rice and sauce. Sprinkle the fish with the remaining ½ teaspoon of salt and the pepper, then spoon a little of the sauce over the fillets.

4. Bake for 15 to 20 minutes, until the fish flakes with a fork.

5. To serve, spoon some rice onto each plate and top with a fillet. Sprinkle with the remaining 1½ teaspoons of parsley.

Thai Curried Halibut with Bok Choy

Prep time: 10 minutes | Cook time: 20 minutes | Serves 4

1 (14-ounce / 397-g) can coconut milk
2 teaspoons red or green Thai curry paste
1 tablespoon fish sauce
1 tablespoon brown sugar
1 tablespoon freshly squeezed lime juice
6 to 8 baby bok choy, trimmed and halved lengthwise
4 (6- to 8-ounce / 170- to 227-g) halibut fillets
¼ cup chopped fresh cilantro

1. Select Bake and preheat the oven to 400ºF (205ºC).

2. Pour the coconut milk into a 9-by-13-inch baking dish, and put the dish in the oven while it preheats.

3. When the coconut milk just begins to simmer, stir in the curry paste, fish sauce, brown sugar, and lime juice.

4. Place the bok choy halves in a single layer in the baking dish and arrange the halibut fillets on top. Spoon some of the coconut milk mixture over the top of the fish.

5. Bake for about 20 minutes, until the halibut flakes with a fork and the bok choy is tender.

Broiled Lemony Salmon Steak

Prep time: 10 minutes | Cook time: 20 minutes | Serves 2

2 (6-ounce / 170-g) salmon steaks
Brushing Mixture:
2 tablespoons lemon juice
2 tablespoons olive oil
1 tablespoon soy sauce
1 teaspoon dried dill or dill weed
½ teaspoon garlic powder
1 teaspoon soy sauce

1. Combine the brushing mixture ingredients in a small bowl and brush the salmon steak tops, skin side down, liberally, reserving the remaining mixture.

Let the steaks sit at room temperature for 10 minutes, then place on a broiling rack with a pan underneath.

2. Broil 15 minutes, remove from the oven, and brush the steaks with the remaining mixture. Broil again for 5 minutes, or until the meat flakes easily with a fork.

Stuffed Tilapia with Pepper and Cucumber

Prep time: 15 minutes | Cook time: 20 minutes | Makes 6 tilapia rolls

6 (5-ounce / 142-g) tilapia fillets
2 tablespoons olive oil

Filling:

1 cucumber, peeled, seeds scooped out and discarded, and chopped
½ cup chopped roasted peppers, drained
2 tablespoons lemon juice
2 tablespoons chopped fresh parsley or cilantro
1 teaspoon garlic powder
1 teaspoon paprika
Salt and freshly ground black pepper, to taste

Dip Mixture:

1 cup nonfat sour cream
2 tablespoons low-fat mayonnaise
3 tablespoons Dijon mustard
1 teaspoon Worcestershire sauce
1 teaspoon dried dill

1. Combine the filling ingredients in a bowl, adjusting the seasonings to taste.
2. Spoon equal portions of filling in the centers of the tilapia filets. Roll up the fillets, starting at the smallest end. Secure each roll with toothpicks and place the rolls in an oiled or nonstick baking pan. Carefully brush the fillets with oil and place them in an oiled or nonstick 8½ × 8½ × 2-inch square baking (cake) pan.
3. Broil for 20 minutes, or until the fillets are lightly browned. Combine the dip mixture ingredients in a small bowl and serve with the fish.

Marinated Catfish Fillet

Prep time: 10 minutes | Cook time: 15 minutes | Serves 4

4 (6-ounce / 170-g) catfish fillets

Marinade Ingredients:

1 tablespoon olive oil
1 tablespoon lemon juice
¼ dry white wine
1 tablespoon garlic powder
1 tablespoon soy sauce

1. Combine the marinade ingredients in an 8½ × 8½ × 4-inch ovenproof baking dish. Add the fillets and let stand for 10 minutes, spooning the marinade over the fillets every 2 minutes.
2. Broil the fillets for 15 minutes, or until the fish flakes easily with a fork.

Fish Fillet with Poblano Sauce

Prep time: 10 minutes | Cook time: 20 minutes | Makes 4 fillets

4 (5-ounce / 142-g) thin fish fillets—perch, scrod, catfish, or flounder
1 tablespoon olive oil

Poblano Sauce:

1 poblano chili, seeded and chopped
1 bell pepper, seeded and chopped
2 tablespoons chopped onion
5 garlic cloves, peeled
1 tablespoon flour
1 cup fat-free half-and-half
Salt, to taste

1. Preheat the toaster oven to 350ºF (180ºC).
2. Brush the fillets with olive oil and transfer to an oiled or nonstick 8½ × 8½ × 2-inch square baking (cake) pan. Set aside.
3. Combine the poblano sauce ingredients and process in a blender or food processor until smooth. Spoon the poblano sauce over the fillets, covering them well.
4. Bake, uncovered, for 20 minutes, or until the fish flakes easily with a fork.

Mediterranean Baked Fish Fillet

Prep time: 10 minutes | Cook time: 25 minutes | Serves 4

4 (6-ounce / 170-g) fish fillets (red snapper, cod, whiting, sole, or mackerel)

Mixture Ingredients:
1 tablespoon olive oil
2 tablespoons tomato paste
3 plum tomatoes, chopped
2 garlic cloves, minced
2 tablespoons capers
2 tablespoons pitted and chopped black olives
2 tablespoons chopped fresh basil leaves
2 tablespoons chopped fresh parsley

1. Preheat the toaster oven to 350ºF (180ºC).
2. Combine the baking mixture ingredients in a small bowl. Set aside.
3. Layer the fillets in an oiled or nonstick 8½ × 8½ × 2-inch square baking (cake) pan, overlapping them if necessary, and spoon the baking mixture over the fish.
4. Bake, covered, for 25 minutes, or until the fish flakes easily with a fork.

Crispy Fish Fillet

Prep time: 10 minutes | Cook time: 14 minutes | Serves 4

4 (6-ounce / 170-g) fish fillets, approximately ¼- to ½-inch thick
2 tablespoons vegetable oil
Coating Ingredients:
1 cup cornmeal
1 teaspoon garlic powder
1 teaspoon ground cumin
1 teaspoon paprika
Salt, to taste

1. Combine the coating ingredients in a small bowl, blending well. Transfer to a large plate, spreading evenly over the surface. Brush the fillets with vegetable oil and press both sides of each fillet into the coating.
2. Broil an oiled or nonstick 8½ × 8½ × 2-inch square baking (cake) pan for 1 or 2 minutes to preheat. Remove the pan and place the fillets in the hot pan, laying them flat.
3. Broil for 7 minutes, then remove the pan from the oven and carefully turn the fillets with a spatula. Broil for another 7 minutes, or until the fish flakes easily with a fork and the coating is crisped to your preference. Serve immediately.

Flounder Fillet and Asparagus Rolls

Prep time: 10 minutes | Cook time: 30 minutes | Serves 4

1 dozen asparagus stalks, tough stem part cut off
4 (6-ounce / 170-g) flounder fillets
4 tablespoons chopped scallions
4 tablespoons shredded carrots
4 tablespoons finely chopped
Almonds
1 teaspoon dried dill weed
Salt and freshly ground black pepper, to taste
1 lemon, cut into wedges

1. Preheat the toaster oven to 400ºF (205ºC).
2. Place 3 asparagus stalks lengthwise on a flounder fillet. Add 1 tablespoon scallions, 1 tablespoon carrots, 1 tablespoon almonds, and a sprinkling of dill. Season to taste with salt and pepper and roll the fillet together so that the long edges overlap. Secure the edges with toothpicks or tie with cotton string. Carefully place the rolled fillet in an oiled or nonstick 8½ × 8½ × 2-inch square baking (cake) pan. Repeat the process for the remaining ingredients. Cover the pan with aluminum foil.
3. Bake, covered, for 20 minutes, or until the asparagus is tender. Remove the cover.
4. Broil, uncovered, for 10 minutes, or until the fish is lightly browned. Remove and discard the toothpicks or string. Serve the rolled fillets with lemon wedges.

Fish Fillet with Sun-Dried Tomato Pesto

Prep time: 10 minutes | Cook time: 31 minutes | Serves 4

4 (6-ounce / 170-g) fish fillets (trout, catfish, flounder, or tilapia)
1 tablespoon reduced-fat mayonnaise
2 tablespoons chopped fresh cilantro Olive oil
Tomato Sauce:
¼ cup chopped sun-dried tomatoes
2 tablespoons chopped fresh basil
$^{2}/_{3}$ cup dry white wine

2 tablespoons grated Parmesan cheese
2 tablespoons olive oil
1 tablespoon pine nuts
2 garlic cloves
Salt and freshly ground black pepper, to taste

1. Preheat the toaster oven to 400ºF (205ºC).
2. Process the tomato sauce ingredients in a blender or food processor until smooth.
3. Layer the fish fillets in an oiled or nonstick 8½ × 8½ × 2-inch square baking (cake) pan. Spoon the sauce over the fish, spreading evenly.
4. Bake, uncovered, for 25 minutes, or until the fish flakes easily with a fork. Remove from the oven, spread the mayonnaise on top of the fish, and garnish with the cilantro.
5. Broil for 6 minutes, or until lightly browned.

Catfish, Toamto and Onion Kebabs

Prep time: 10 minutes | Cook time: 20 minutes | Serves 4

4 (5-ounce / 142-g) catfish fillets
4 (9-inch) metal skewers
2 plum tomatoes, quartered
1 onion, cut into 1 × 1-inch pieces

Marinade:

3 tablespoons lemon juice
3 tablespoons tomato juice
2 garlic cloves, minced
2 tablespoons olive oil
1 teaspoon soy sauce

1. Combine the marinade ingredients in a small bowl. Set aside.
2. Cut the fillets into 2 by 3-inch strips and place in a shallow glass or ceramic dish. Add the marinade and refrigerate, covered, for at least 20 minutes. Remove the strips from the marinade, roll, and skewer, alternating the rolled strips with the tomatoes and onion.
3. Brush the kebabs with marinade, reserving the remaining marinade for brushing again later. Place the skewers on a broiling rack with a pan underneath.
4. Broil for 10 minutes, then remove the pan from the oven and carefully turn the skewers. Brush the kebabs with the marinade and broil again for 10 minutes, or until browned.

CHAPTER 5 VEGETABLES

Goat Cheese and Roasted Red Pepper Tarts

Prep time: 10 minutes | Cook time: 1¼ hours | Serves 4 to 6

4 red bell peppers, seeded, stemmed, and halved
4 tablespoons olive oil, divided
4 ounces (113 g) fresh goat cheese, divided
$^{1}/_{3}$ cup heavy (whipping) cream
All-purpose flour, for dusting
1 sheet frozen puff pastry, thawed according to package directions
Kosher salt, to taste
Freshly ground black pepper, to taste
2 teaspoons chopped fresh oregano leaves, divided
1 large egg, beaten

1. Select Bake and preheat the oven to 425ºF (220ºC).
2. Place a rack in the upper third of the oven. Line a baking sheet with parchment paper.
3. Arrange the bell peppers, cut-side down, on the prepared sheet and drizzle with 2 tablespoons of olive oil. Bake for about 40 minutes, until the peppers are tender and the skins begin to blacken. Transfer to a bowl, cover with plastic wrap, and let steam for 10 to 15 minutes. Slip off the skins and cut the peppers into thin strips.
4. While the peppers roast, whisk until smooth 2 ounces of goat cheese and the heavy cream in a small bowl.
5. On a lightly floured board, roll the pastry sheet out to an 11-by-17-inch rectangle (if your oven won't fit such a large pan, make two smaller rectangles instead of one and bake on two baking sheets). Transfer the pastry to the prepared sheet.
6. Spread the goat cheese–cream mixture over the pastry, leaving a 1-inch border all the way around.
7. Arrange the sliced bell peppers over the cream and crumble the remaining 2 ounces of goat cheese over the top.
8. Season with salt and pepper and drizzle with the remaining 2 tablespoons of olive oil. Sprinkle the oregano over the top.
9. Brush the pastry border with the beaten egg. Bake for about 10 minutes, until the pastry begins to puff up and brown lightly. Lower the oven temperature to 375ºF (190ºC) and bake for 15 to 20 minutes more, until the pastry is deep golden brown and cooked through. Serve warm or at room temperature.

Double Cheese Corn and Chard Gratin

Prep time: 15 minutes | Cook time: 35 minutes | Serves 4 to 6

Nonstick cooking spray, for preparing the baking dish
½ teaspoon kosher salt, plus more for salting the water and seasoning
1 pound (454 g) chard, stemmed
2 tablespoons olive oil, divided
2 garlic cloves, minced
1 teaspoon chopped fresh rosemary leaves
1 teaspoon fresh thyme leaves
Freshly ground black pepper, to taste
3 large eggs
½ cup half-and-half
2 cups corn kernels (from 2 to 3 ears, or use thawed frozen corn)
1 cup shredded Gruyère cheese
¼ cup freshly grated Parmesan cheese

1. Select Bake and preheat the oven to 375ºF (190ºC).
2. Spray an 8- or 9-inch square baking dish with cooking spray. Fill a large bowl with ice water.
3. Bring a large pot of salted water to a boil over high heat. Blanch the chard leaves in the boiling water for 1 to 2 minutes, until tender but still bright green. Transfer to the ice-water bath to stop the cooking. Drain well. Squeeze out any excess water and chop the leaves.
4. In a medium skillet over medium heat, heat 1 tablespoon of olive oil.
5. Add the garlic. Cook for 30 seconds to 1 minute, stirring, until fragrant.
6. Stir in the rosemary, thyme, and chopped blanched chard. Season with salt and pepper. Cook

for about 1 minute, stirring, until the chard is nicely coated with oil. Remove from the heat.

7. In a large bowl, whisk the eggs, half-and-half, and remaining ½ teaspoon of salt.

8. Add the chard, corn, and Gruyère. Stir to mix well. Transfer the mixture to the prepared baking dish and sprinkle the Parmesan over the top.

9. Drizzle with the remaining 1 tablespoon of olive oil. Bake for 30 to 35 minutes, until the top is bubbling and nicely browned. Remove from the oven and let it rest for 5 to 10 minutes before serving.

Feta Zucchini Fritters with Garlicky Yogurt

Prep time: 15 minutes | Cook time: 20 minutes | Serves 4 to 6

For the Fritters:

2 zucchini, grated on the large holes of a box grater
½ teaspoon kosher salt
2 garlic cloves, minced
1 tablespoon olive oil
1 teaspoon baking powder
¼ teaspoon freshly ground black pepper
2 large eggs
¾ cup crumbled Feta cheese
1 cup panko bread crumbs
2 scallions, white and green parts, thinly sliced

For the Dipping Sauce:

1 cup nonfat Greek yogurt
2 garlic cloves, minced
2 tablespoons chopped fresh dill leaves
1 tablespoon freshly squeezed lemon juice
½ teaspoon kosher salt

Make the Fritters

1. Select Bake and preheat the oven to 375ºF (190ºC).

2. Line a baking sheet with parchment paper.

3. Put the grated zucchini in a colander and toss with the salt. Let drain over the sink for 5 to 10 minutes. Press on the zucchini to squeeze out as much liquid as you can. Transfer to a large bowl.

4. To the zucchini, add the garlic, olive oil, baking powder, pepper, eggs, Feta cheese, and bread crumbs. Stir to combine. Scoop or spoon the mixture, using about 2 tablespoons per fritter, onto the prepared sheet. Bake for 18 to 20 minutes, until the fritters are crisp and golden on the outside. Let cool for a few minutes before serving warm with the yogurt sauce for dipping.

Make the Dipping Sauce

5. While the fritters bake, stir together the yogurt, garlic, dill, lemon juice, and salt in a small bowl.

Balsamic Prosciutto-Wrapped Asparagus

Prep time: 5 minutes | Cook time: 10 minutes | Serves 4

6 to 8 (4-ounce / 113-g) thin slices Prosciutto di Parma or serrano ham
1 pound (454 g) asparagus, trimmed
2 teaspoons aged balsamic vinegar

1. Select Bake and preheat the oven to 375ºF (190ºC).

2. Cut the prosciutto into long strips (one strip per asparagus spear). Starting at the bottom of the spear, wrap each piece of asparagus about halfway to two-thirds of the way up with a strip of prosciutto, wrapping at an angle. Place the wrapped spears on a sheet pan.

3. Bake the asparagus for 10 to 12 minutes, until the asparagus is tender and the prosciutto is crisp. Very thick spears may take longer.

4. Transfer the asparagus to a platter. Drizzle with the balsamic vinegar. Serve warm or at room temperature.

Chives Stuffed Baked Potatoes

Prep time: 10 minutes | Cook time: 58 minutes | Serves 4

2 large baking potatoes, slit on top with a knife
⅛ teaspoon paprika
Salt and freshly ground black pepper, to taste

For the Stuffing:

1 teaspoon margarine
1 egg, lightly beaten
½ cup nonfat sour cream
4 tablespoons fresh or frozen and thawed chives

1. Preheat the toaster oven to 400ºF (205ºC).

2. Bake the potatoes on the oven rack for 50 minutes, or until tender. Open the slits with a knife

and scoop out the pulp with a teaspoon. Set the potato shells aside.

3. Combine the stuffing ingredients and add the pulp, mixing well, until light and fluffy. Refill the potato shells.

4. Broil 8 minutes, or until the top is lightly browned. Sprinkle with the chives before serving.

Golden Potato, Carrot and Onion

Prep time: 10 minutes | Cook time: 38 minutes | Serves 4

2 cups peeled and shredded potatoes
½ cup peeled and shredded carrots
¼ cup shredded onion
1 teaspoon salt
1 teaspoon dried rosemary
1 teaspoon dried cumin
3 tablespoons vegetable oil
Salt and freshly ground black pepper, to taste

1. Preheat the toaster oven to 400ºF (205ºC).
2. Mix all the ingredients together in a 1-quart 8½ × 8½ × 2-inch ovenproof baking dish. Adjust the seasonings to taste. Cover the dish with aluminum foil.
3. Bake, covered, for 30 minutes, or until tender. Remove the cover.
4. Broil for 8 minutes, or until the top is browned.

Potato Shells with Cheddar and Bacon

Prep time: 5 minutes | Cook time: 8 minutes | Serves 4

4 tablespoons shredded reduced-fat Cheddar cheese
4 slices lean turkey bacon, cooked and crumbled
4 potato shells
4 tablespoons nonfat sour cream
4 teaspoons chopped fresh or frozen chives
Salt and freshly ground black pepper, to taste

1. Sprinkle 1 tablespoon Cheddar cheese and 1 tablespoon crumbled bacon into each potato shell. Place the shells on a broiling rack with a pan underneath.
2. Broil for 8 minutes, or until the cheese is melted and the shells lightly browned. Spoon 1 tablespoon sour cream into each shell and sprinkle with 1 teaspoon chives. Add salt and pepper to taste.

Ranch Barbecue Potatoes

Prep time: 5 minutes | Cook time: 50 minutes | Serves 2

2 medium russet potatoes, scrubbed and cut lengthwise into ¼-inch strips
1 medium onion, chopped
2 tablespoons vegetable oil
2 tablespoons barbecue sauce
¼ teaspoon hot sauce
Salt and freshly ground black pepper, to taste

1. Preheat the toaster oven to 400ºF (205ºC).
2. Combine all the ingredients in a medium bowl, mixing well and adjusting the seasonings to taste.
3. Place equal portions of the potatoes on two 12 × 12-inch squares of heavy-duty aluminum foil. Fold up the edges of the foil to form a sealed packet and place on the oven rack.
4. Bake for 40 minutes, or until the potatoes are tender. Carefully open the packet and fold back the foil.
5. Broil 10 minutes, or until the potatoes are browned.

Garlicky Potatoes

Prep time: 5 minutes | Cook time: 50 minutes | Serves 2

2 medium potatoes, peeled and chopped
6 garlic cloves, roasted
1 tablespoon olive oil
Salt and freshly ground black pepper, to taste
1 tablespoon chopped fresh parsley

1. Preheat the toaster oven to 400ºF (205ºC).
2. Place the potatoes in an oiled or nonstick 8½ × 8½ × 2-inch square baking (cake) pan. Add the garlic, oil, and salt and pepper to taste. Toss to coat well. Cover the pan with aluminum foil.
3. Bake, covered, for 40 minutes, or until the potatoes are tender. Remove the cover.
4. Broil 10 minutes, or until lightly browned. Garnish with fresh parsley before serving.

Baked Garlic Buds

Prep time: 5 minutes | Cook time: 20 minutes | Makes ¾ cup

3 whole garlic buds
3 tablespoons olive oil
Salt and freshly ground black pepper, to taste

1. Preheat the toaster oven to 450ºF (235ºC).
2. Place the garlic buds in an oiled or nonstick 8½ × 8½ × 2-inch square baking (cake) pan.
3. Bake, uncovered, for 20 minutes, or until the buds are tender when pierced with a skewer or sharp knife. When cool enough to handle, peel and mash the baked cloves with a fork into the olive oil. Season with salt and pepper to taste.

Classic Cornucopia Casserole

Prep time: 15 minutes | Cook time: 45 minutes | Serves 4

1 celery stalk, chopped
2 tablespoons chopped Vidalia onion
3½ bell pepper, chopped
1 carrot, peeled and chopped
1 small zucchini, chopped
½ cup green beans, cut into 1-inch Pieces
½ cup frozen peas
½ cup frozen corn
½ cup frozen broccoli florets
½ cup frozen cauliflower florets
2 tablespoons vegetable oil
1 teaspoon ground cumin
1 teaspoon garlic powder
½ teaspoon paprika
Salt and freshly ground black pepper, to taste
½ cup finely chopped pecans
3 tablespoons grated Parmesan cheese

1. Preheat the toaster oven to 400ºF (205ºC).
2. Combine all the ingredients, except the pecans and Parmesan cheese, in a 1-quart 8½ × 8½ × 4-inch ovenproof baking dish and adjust the seasonings to taste. Cover with aluminum foil.
3. Bake, covered, for 35 minutes, or until the vegetables are tender. Uncover, stir to distribute the liquid, and adjust the seasonings again. Sprinkle the top with the pecans and Parmesan cheese.
4. Broil for 10 minutes, or until the pecans are lightly browned.

Parmesan Tomato Casserole

Prep time: 10 minutes | Cook time: 45 minutes | Serves 4

1 medium onion, coarsely chopped
3 medium tomatoes, coarsely chopped
1 medium green pepper, coarsely chopped
2 garlic cloves, minced
½ teaspoon crushed oregano
½ teaspoon crushed basil
1 tablespoon extra-virgin olive oil
2 tablespoons chopped fresh cilantro
Salt and freshly ground black pepper, to taste
3 to 4 tablespoons grated Parmesan cheese
¼ cup multigrain bread crumbs

1. Preheat the toaster oven to 400ºF (205ºC).
2. Combine the casserole mixture ingredients in a 1-quart 8½ × 8½ × 4-inch ovenproof baking dish. Adjust the seasonings to taste and cover with aluminum foil.
3. Bake, covered, for 35 minutes, or until the tomatoes and pepper are tender. Remove from the oven, uncover, and sprinkle with the bread crumbs and Parmesan cheese.
4. Broil for 10 minutes, or until the topping is lightly browned.

Roasted Beans and Tomatoes with Tahini

Prep time: 15 minutes | Cook time: 20 minutes | Serves 6

For the Vegetables:

1 pound (454 g) cherry tomatoes, mixed colors if possible
2 tablespoons extra-virgin olive oil
Sea salt flakes and freshly ground black pepper, to taste
1 pound (454 g) string beans, stem ends removed
1½ teaspoons cumin seeds
2 teaspoons sesame seeds
2 tablespoons roughly chopped cilantro leaves

For the Tahini Dressing:

¼ cup tahini

Juice of ½ lemon
5 tablespoons water, plus more if needed
2 garlic cloves, finely grated
4 tablespoons extra-virgin olive oil
1½ teaspoons clear honey

1. Preheat the oven to 400ºF (205ºC).
2. Put the tomatoes into a bake pan or on a baking sheet that has a lip all the way around. There needs to be room to add the beans later. Toss the tomatoes with 1 tablespoon of the oil and season them well. Roast in the oven for 10 minutes.
3. Toss the string beans in a bowl with the remaining 1 tablespoon of oil and the cumin seeds. Scatter the beans on top and around the tomatoes. Return to the oven for a final 10 minutes. At the end of the roasting time, the tomatoes should be completely soft and the beans slightly charred.
4. To make the dressing, mix all the ingredients together in a bowl and season well. The tahini will "seize" and thicken when you add the lemon juice, but don't worry, it will break down again when you add the water and beat hard with a wooden spoon. Tahini varies in thickness, so you might need more water than I've suggested here to achieve a dressing as thick as cream.
5. Spoon the dressing onto a plate, place the vegetables on top, and scatter with the sesame seeds and cilantro. You can serve this at room temperature, though I prefer it slightly warm.

Spiced Date Buttered Eggplant

Prep time: 15 minutes | Cook time: 40 minutes | Serves 6

For the Butter:

Good pinch of saffron threads
6 black cardamom pods
4 tablespoons unsalted butter, at room temperature
4 Medjool dates, pitted and chopped
2 garlic cloves, crushed
¼ teaspoon cayenne pepper, or to taste
Generous pinch of ground ginger, or to taste
Sea salt flakes, to taste

For the Eggplants:

6¾ pounds (3.1 kg) globe eggplants
A little extra-virgin olive oil
Black sesame seeds, to serve
Plain yogurt, to serve

1. Preheat the oven to 400ºF (205ºC).
2. For the butter, put the saffron into a small bowl or cup and add ½ tablespoon boiling water. Stir, then leave to cool. Break the cardamom pods open and remove the seeds. Grind them as well as you can with a mortar and pestle.
3. Put the butter into a bowl, add the saffron and cardamom, and stir and mash to combine well. Add the dates, garlic, cayenne, and ginger, and season well with salt. Stir and mash to combine again, then taste: you may want more cayenne or ginger, but these spices shouldn't overwhelm the cardamom. Shape the butter into a log and wrap it in parchment paper, or just transfer it to a bowl and cover it. Either way, it needs to go into the refrigerator (because of the dates, this is better a little chilled).
4. Put the eggplants in a bake pan and brush lightly with some of the oil. Pierce each one a few times with the tines of a fork. Bake for 40 to 45 minutes, or until the eggplants are completely soft and look a bit deflated.
5. Slit the eggplants down the middle. Add pats of the spiced date butter and allow them to melt. Sprinkle on sesame seeds, and serve with a bowl of yogurt.

Greek Feta Zucchini Pie

Prep time: 10 minutes | Cook time: 35 minutes | Serves 4

2¼ pounds (1 kg) zucchini, cut into ¾in thick slices
3 tablespoons extra-virgin olive oil
Sea salt flakes and freshly ground black pepper, to taste
8 thin scallions, trimmed
5 large eggs, lightly beaten
$^{2}/_{3}$ cup Greek yogurt
Scant ¼ cup instant polenta
Scant 1 cup crumbled Feta cheese
1 cup finely grated kefalotyri or pecorino cheese
¼ cup chopped dill leaves, any thick stalks discarded, plus more to serve
3 garlic cloves, finely grated

1. Preheat the oven to 400ºF (205ºC).
2. Put the zucchini into a large bake pan in which they can lie—more or less—in a single layer. Toss them with 2 tablespoons of the olive oil and season. Bake for 10 minutes, then add the scallions

and trickle the remaining 1 tablespoon of oil over them. Return to the oven and bake for another 10 to 15 minutes. By this time, the zucchini should be tender when pierced with a sharp knife, and the scallions slightly charred.

3. Reduce the oven temperature to 350ºF (180ºC).

4. In a large bowl, mix together all the other ingredients and season well. Spoon the vegetables into a gratin dish; mine measures 10½ x 8 x 2in and has a capacity of 1 quart. A cast-iron or tin-lined copper dish is best, because the metals conduct heat well. Pour the batter over the vegetables and bake in the oven for 15 to 20 minutes, or until just set, golden, and slightly souffléd. Serve hot or warm, scattered with dill.

Chili Tomato with Herbs and Pistachios

Prep time: 15 minutes | Cook time: 30 minutes | Serves

1²/₃ pounds (756 g) plum tomatoes, halved lengthwise
4 tablespoons extra-virgin olive oil
3 teaspoons crushed red pepper
2 teaspoons fennel seeds
Sea salt flakes and freshly ground black pepper, to taste
4 teaspoons clear honey
1 cup Greek yogurt, or more, depending on the size of your serving plate
1 cup crumbled Feta cheese
1 garlic clove, finely grated
¹/₃ cup dill, chopped, any thick stalks removed
Scant 1 cup mint leaves
1 tablespoon chopped shelled unsalted pistachio nuts

1. Preheat the oven to 400ºF (205ºC).

2. Put all the tomatoes into a bake pan in which they can lie in a single layer; if they are too close to each other, they will steam instead of roasting. Spoon 3 tablespoons of the oil over them, then turn them over with your hands so they get well coated. Leave them cut sides up.

3. Put the crushed red pepper and fennel seeds into a mortar and bash them. You won't break the fennel seeds down, but you'll crush them a bit. Sprinkle these over the tomatoes and season. Mix the honey with the remaining olive oil and spoon a little over each tomato.

4. Cook for 30 minutes. Keep an eye on them; you may find they need a little longer, but don't overcook them. They get to a point when they completely collapse and even though they're delicious at this stage, they've lost all their shape and you don't want that here.

5. Stir the yogurt, Feta, and garlic together and season. Put the yogurt mixture on a serving plate and pile the roast tomatoes on top. Sprinkle the herbs and pistachios all over the dish and serve.

Lemony-Honey Roasted Radishes

Prep time: 10 minutes | Cook time: 17 minutes | Serves 4

1 pound (454 g) radishes, with green leaves attached
1 tablespoon extra-virgin olive oil
1 tablespoon white balsamic vinegar
1 preserved lemon, flesh discarded, rind cut into shreds, plus 2 tablespoons brine from the jar, plus more if needed
1 tablespoon unsalted butter
Sea salt flakes and freshly ground black pepper, to taste
1½ tablespoons clear honey
Leaves from 6 mint sprigs, torn

1. Preheat the oven to 400ºF (205ºC).

2. Wash the radishes well and remove their leaves (keep them fresh: you can wrap them in damp paper towels and put them in the refrigerator).

3. Halve the radishes lengthwise. Put them in a bake pan with the olive oil, white balsamic, half the preserved lemon brine, and all the butter. Season. Bake for 7 minutes.

4. Add the remaining tablespoon of brine and the honey. Shake the pan around and return to the oven for a final 10 minutes.

5. Transfer to a warmed serving dish and mix in the reserved radish leaves; they will wilt in the heat. Stir in the shredded preserved lemon rind and taste for seasoning (you might want a little more of the brine). Scatter on the mint leaves and serve.

Stuffed Peppers with Cheese and Basil

Prep time: 10 minutes | Cook time: 40 minutes | Serves 6

6 medium bell peppers
A little extra-virgin olive oil
5½ ounces (156 g) ricotta (fresh rather than ultra-pasteurized, if possible)
10½ ounces (297.7 g) soft goat cheese
1 cup finely grated Parmesan cheese
Sea salt flakes and freshly ground black pepper, to taste
1 cup basil leaves, torn
1 large egg
1 garlic clove, crushed
1 tablespoon toasted pine nuts (optional)

1. Preheat the oven to 375ºF (190ºC).
2. Halve the peppers, deseed them, brush them with olive oil, and put them into a gratin dish from which they can be served.
3. Drain the ricotta and the goat cheese (there can be a little moisture lying on top of them). Mix together all three cheeses with seasoning, the basil, egg, and garlic, gently mashing. Add the pine nuts if you are using them.
4. Spoon the mixture into the pepper halves and bake for 40 minutes. The filling should be golden and souffléd and the peppers completely tender when pierced with a sharp knife. If they're not ready, return them to the oven for an extra 5 to 10 minutes, then test again.

Moroccan Roasted Veggies with Labneh

Prep time: 20 minutes | Cook time: 40 minutes | Serves 6

For the Labneh:

¾ cup Greek yogurt
Sea salt flakes and freshly ground black pepper, to taste

For the Vegetables:

4½ pounds (2 kg) winter squash or pumpkin
3 onions, cut into thick wedges
2 pounds (907 g) cauliflower florets
1 pound (454 g) creamer potatoes, scrubbed and quartered
2 to 3 red Fresno chilies, halved, seeded, and thinly sliced
1¼-inch fresh ginger, peeled and finely grated
½ tablespoon ground cumin
1 tablespoon harissa
7 tablespoons extra-virgin olive oil
2 (15-ounce / 425-g) cans of chickpeas, drained and rinsed
4 garlic cloves, finely sliced
½ pound (227 g) cherry tomatoes
Juice of ½ lemon
½ cup chopped cilantro leaves, to serve
3 preserved lemons, rind only, shredded, to serve
Couscous, to serve (optional)

1. Start the labneh the day before. Put the yogurt into a piece of cheesecloth or a brand new all-purpose kitchen cloth set in a sieve over a bowl. Stir in some salt and pepper. Pull the fabric up round the yogurt to make a "bag." Put the whole thing, including the bowl to catch the liquid that drains out in the refrigerator for 24 hours. Give it a gentle squeeze every so often. You'll get a firm yogurt "cheese."
2. Preheat the oven to 400ºF (205ºC).
3. Cut the squash into wedges (I don't peel it, as the skin softens enough during roasting to be edible) and remove the seeds. Divide between 2 bake pans, then do the same with the onions, cauliflower, and potatoes. The vegetables need to be able to lie in a single layer, with room to add the tomatoes later. Season, add the chilies, ginger, cumin, and harissa, and drizzle everything with 5 tablespoons of the olive oil. Turn the vegetables so they get covered in the flavorings and oil. Bake for 20 minutes.
4. Stir in the chickpeas and garlic, add the tomatoes, and drizzle with the rest of the olive oil. Bake for a final 20 minutes, or until the vegetables are tender and slightly charred in places. Check the seasoning.
5. Transfer the vegetables to a warmed platter or shallow bowl. Squeeze over the lemon juice and scatter with the cilantro and shredded preserved lemon rind. Serve the vegetables and labneh on their own, the dish already contains a starch in the potatoes or with couscous.

Oregano Eggplants with Chili Anchovy Sauce

Prep time: 15 minutes | Cook time: 40 minutes | Serves 4

For the Eggplants:

4¾ pounds (2.2 g) globe eggplants
4 tablespoons extra-virgin olive oil
Leaves from 3 oregano sprigs, torn
Sea salt flakes and freshly ground black pepper, to taste
Juice of ½ lemon
Good crusty bread, to serve

For the Sauce:

Leaves from 2 rosemary sprigs
2 garlic cloves, chopped
14 anchovies, drained of oil
Juice of 1 lemon, or to taste
4 tablespoons extra-virgin olive oil
1 red Fresno chili, halved, seeded, and chopped, plus more if you want it hotter

1. Preheat the oven to 400ºF (205ºC).
2. Halve the eggplants and cut a cross-hatched pattern in the flesh of each one, without cutting all the way through to the skin (this helps the heat to penetrate better). Put them on to a rimmed baking sheet—line it with parchment paper or foil if you want and smear the olive oil evenly all over the cut surfaces. Toss in the oregano, too, and salt and pepper. Turn the eggplants over with your hands, making sure the seasoning and some of the herb leaves go into the flesh.
3. Bake, cut side up, for about 40 minutes, or until the eggplants are completely tender right through and golden. Squeeze the lemon juice over the top.
4. To make the sauce, pound the rosemary and garlic in a mortar, then add the anchovies and crush to a paste. Gradually add the lemon juice and then the olive oil, a little at a time, grinding as you go. You aren't making a mayonnaise—so don't expect this to emulsify, you'll be left with a lumpy "sauce"—but the pounding melds all the elements together. Add the chili and set aside. The longer the sauce sits with the chili, the hotter it will become.
5. Serve the eggplants with the sauce, either on the side or spooned over the top. You need good bread with this, to mop up all the juices.

Parmesan Fennel with Red Pepper

Prep time: 10 minutes | Cook time: 30 minutes | Serves 6 to 8

4 fennel bulbs
3 tablespoons extra-virgin olive oil
2 garlic cloves, finely grated
3 teaspoons fennel seeds, coarsely crushed in a mortar
3 teaspoons crushed red pepper
Sea salt flakes and freshly ground black pepper, to taste
½ cup finely grated Parmesan cheese

1. Preheat the oven to 400ºF (205ºC).
2. Trim the tips of the fennel bulbs, halve the bulbs and remove any thicker or discolored outer leaves (reserve any little fronds you find). Cut each half into ¾-in thick wedges, keeping them intact at the base. Toss in a bowl with the olive oil, garlic, fennel seeds, crushed red pepper, any reserved fennel fronds, and plenty of seasoning. Put into a gratin dish and cover tightly with foil.
3. Bake for about 20 minutes (the undersides should turn pale gold), then remove the foil, sprinkle on the Parmesan, and return to the oven for a final 10 to 15 minutes, or until the fennel is tender (check it by piercing a piece with a sharp knife) and the top is golden.

Buttery Eggplant and Tomato with Freekeh

Prep time: 20 minutes | Cook time: 30 minutes | Serves 4

For the Vegetables and Freekeh:

2¼ pounds (1 kg) baby eggplants
2¼ pounds (1 kg) plum tomatoes
7 tablespoons unsalted butter
12 garlic cloves, thickly sliced
Sea salt flakes and freshly ground black pepper, to taste

A little light brown sugar (optional, only if your tomatoes aren't sweet)
Scant 2 cups cooked freekeh
Plain yogurt, to serve
Good bread, to serve

For the Koch-Kocha:

½ green bell pepper, halved, seeded, and roughly chopped
4 cups cilantro leaves
1 red Fresno chili and 1 green chili, halved and deseeded
1¼-inch fresh ginger, peeled and finely grated
Juice of 1 lime
½ tablespoon cider vinegar or white wine vinegar
1 garlic clove, finely grated
1 teaspoon ground cumin
1 teaspoon ground cardamom
¼ teaspoon grains of paradise, crushed
½ teaspoon ajwain, crushed
7 tablespoons extra-virgin olive oil

1. Preheat the oven to 400ºF (205ºC).
2. Pierce each eggplant with the tip of a knife, you don't have to remove the tops and cut the tomatoes in half. Put them into a bake pan or a shallow casserole 12-in in diameter; they don't have to quite lie in a single layer but they should almost do so.
3. Melt the butter in a saucepan and add the garlic. Cook over a low heat for a few minutes, then pour the butter all over the vegetables, turning them over. Season and sprinkle each tomato half with a little sugar if they aren't very sweet; if you have great tomatoes you won't need it.
4. Bake for 30 minutes, turning the eggplants over once during this time.
5. For the koch-kocha sauce, simply put everything into a food processor and whizz until smooth.
6. Add the freekeh to the bake pan, pushing it down under the vegetables (you don't want it sprinkled on top of them). Return to the oven for a final 5 to 10 minutes, or until the tomatoes are caramelized, the eggplants are tender right through, and the freekeh has become slightly sticky at the edges. Serve the dish with the sauce, a big bowl of plain yogurt, and good bread.

Cheesy Eggplant with Chili Smoked Almonds

Prep time: 10 minutes | Cook time: 45 minutes | Serves 6

3¾ pounds (1.7 kg) globe eggplants
5 tablespoons extra-virgin olive oil
2 teaspoons harissa
Sea salt flakes and freshly ground black pepper, to taste
2 garlic cloves (not too large), finely grated
Juice of ½ lemon, or to taste
3½ ounces (99.2 g) goat curd or soft creamy goat cheese
1 tablespoon smoked almonds, roughly chopped (you want quite big bits)
2 red Fresno chilies, halved, seeded, and very thinly sliced
Leaves from 1 rosemary sprig, chopped
Warm flatbread or toasted sourdough bread, to serve

1. Preheat the oven to 400ºF (205ºC).
2. Put the eggplants in a bake pan and brush lightly with some of the olive oil. Pierce each a few times with the tines of a fork. Bake for 40 to 45 minutes, or until the eggplants are completely soft and look a bit deflated.
3. Leave until cool enough to handle, then slit the skins and scoop the flesh out into a bowl. Chop the flesh (it will be totally soft, you just need to break it down a bit). Mash, and add about 3½ tablespoons of the oil, the harissa, salt, pepper, garlic, and lemon juice to taste. Put this into a warmed serving bowl and scatter the goat cheese on top.
4. Heat the remaining extra-virgin olive oil in a frying pan and quickly fry the smoked almonds, chilies, and rosemary together (you just want to take the rawness off the chilies a little). Pour this over the roast eggplants and serve with bread.

Smoked Paprika Vegetable with Eggs

Prep time: 15 minutes | Cook time: 41 minutes | Serves 4

4 zucchini

1 pound (454 g) small waxy potatoes, scrubbed and quartered
$^{2}/_{3}$ pound (302.4 g) cherry tomatoes
12 scallions, trimmed
3 tablespoons extra-virgin olive oil
Sea salt flakes and freshly ground black pepper, to taste
Leaves from 3 thyme sprigs, plus 5 whole thyme sprigs
½ teaspoon crushed red pepper (optional)
¾ tablespoon smoked paprika, plus more to serve
4 garlic cloves, finely grated
½ pound (227 g) string beans, stem ends removed
6 to 8 extra-large eggs
Greek yogurt, to serve (optional)

1. Preheat the oven to 400ºF (205ºC).
2. Trim the ends from the zucchini and cut them into ¼in thick slices. Put all the vegetables except the string beans into a shallow casserole, ideally about 12in across, or a bake pan in which they can all lie in a single layer. Add 2 tablespoons of the olive oil, the seasoning, thyme, crushed red pepper (if you want heat), smoked paprika, and garlic. Toss everything together and bake for 30 minutes, turning the vegetables over a couple of times.
3. Toss the string beans with the remaining oil and scatter them on top of the other vegetables. Return to the oven for 8 minutes.
4. Break the eggs on top, season, and return the casserole or pan to the oven for a final 8 minutes or so. The eggs should be cooked.
5. Serve straight from the pan, sprinkling the eggs with a little more paprika, if you like. If you've made it very spicy and I often do a bowl of Greek yogurt on the side is good.

Double Cheese Roasted Asparagus

Prep time: 5 minutes | Cook time: 10 minutes | Serves 4

$^{2}/_{3}$ pound (302.4 g) asparagus spears, of medium thickness
Extra-virgin olive oil
Sea salt flakes and freshly ground black pepper, to taste
4½ ounces (127.6 g) ricotta cheese (fresh rather than ultra-pasteurized, if possible)
Pecorino cheese, or Parmesan cheese, shaved

1. Preheat the oven to 425ºF (220ºC).
2. Trim the woody ends from the asparagus spears, put them on an sheet pan with a slight lip, and drizzle with olive oil. Season with salt.
3. Bake for 10 to 12 minutes, or until the asparagus spears are tender (test one of the thickest with the tip of a sharp knife).
4. Put the asparagus on a serving plate. Scatter the ricotta in nuggets over the top, followed by the shaved pecorino or Parmesan cheese. Season with salt and pepper, pour on more olive oil, and serve immediately.

Tomato and Black Olive Clafoutis

Prep time: 15 minutes | Cook time: 50 minutes | Serves 6

1 pound (454 g) mixed cherry and plum tomatoes, halved or quartered, depending on size
1½ tablespoons extra-virgin olive oil
Sea salt flakes and freshly ground black pepper, to taste
4 large eggs, plus
2 large egg yolks
$^{1}/_{3}$ cup all-purpose flour
Scant 1 cup milk
1¼ cups heavy cream
Generous ½ cup finely grated Parmesan cheese
1 garlic clove, finely grated
2 tablespoons chopped pitted black olives
7 ounces (198 g) soft goat cheese, crumbled
$^{1}/_{3}$ cup basil leaves, torn

1. Preheat the oven to 400ºF (205ºC).
2. Put the tomatoes into a gratin dish with the olive oil and season them. Turn them over so the surfaces are all coated in a little oil. Bake for 20 to 30 minutes, or until the tomatoes are soft and slightly shrunken. Take out of the oven and leave to sit on a work surface.
3. Reduce the oven temperature to 375ºF (190ºC).

4. Put the eggs, egg yolks, flour, milk, and cream into a food processor, season well, and whizz. Stir in the Parmesan and garlic.

5. Scatter the olives over the tomatoes and crumble on the goat cheese.

6. Pour the batter over the tomatoes, olives, and cheese and bake for 30 minutes, until the custard is puffed, golden, and just set in the middle. Leave it for 5 minutes to settle: it will sink a little once it has sat for a while. Scatter over the basil and serve.

Roast Vegetable with Avocado

Prep time: 15 minutes | Cook time: 40 minutes | Serves 4

For the Vegetables:

4 ears of corn

5 zucchini, cut into 3in-long batons

2 red bell peppers, halved, seeded, and cut into broad strips

1 green chili and 2 red Fresno chillies, halved, seeded, and very thinly sliced

1 tablespoon ground cumin

¾ teaspoon ground cinnamon

2 teaspoons dried oregano (preferably Mexican oregano, but regular will do)

4 garlic cloves, finely grated

¼ cup extra-virgin olive oil

Sea salt flakes and freshly ground black pepper, to taste

Scant ½ cup cilantro leaves

To Serve:

2 avocados

Juice of 1 lime, plus lime wedges to serve

$^2/_3$ cup sour cream

3½ ounces (99.2 g) crumbled cheese, such as queso fresco or Feta

Rice, quinoa, or tortillas

1. Preheat the oven to 400ºF (205ºC).

2. Cut the pointed tip off one ear of corn. Hold it standing up in a bake pan. Using a sharp knife, cut down the sides, removing the kernels as you work around. (Try to keep some in strips; cut close to the core to achieve this.) Repeat with the other ears.

3. Put the zucchini and peppers into another bake pan. In a small bowl, mix together the chilies, spices, oregano, garlic, olive oil, and seasoning. Mix two-thirds of this with the zucchini and peppers (reserve the rest of the mixture), tossing with your hands so that all the vegetables get coated.

4. Roast the zucchini and peppers in the oven for 20 minutes, then turn them over. Toss the rest of the oil and spices with the corn, season, and roast that, in its separate pan, alongside the other vegetables for a final 20 minutes.

5. Halve and pit the avocados. Squeeze lime juice all over the surfaces and season. Serve the roasted vegetables in a warmed broad, shallow bowl, scattered with the cilantro leaves, along with the halved avocados, the sour cream, cheese, and lime wedges. Serve rice, quinoa, or tortillas on the side.

Roast Bell Peppers with Burrata and 'Nduja

Prep time: 5 minutes | Cook time: 30 minutes | Serves 4

6 red bell peppers

A little extra-virgin olive oil

Sea salt flakes and freshly ground black pepper, to taste

2¼ ounces (63.8 g) 'nduja

1 pound (454 g) burrata

Ciabatta, to serve

1. Preheat the oven to 400ºF (205ºC).

2. Halve the peppers, seed them, and put them into a gratin dish, bake pan, or a baking sheet with a lip around it. Brush them with olive oil, season, and bake for 20 minutes.

3. Break the 'nduja into chunks and divide it among the peppers, putting it inside them. Bake for a final 10 minutes.

4. When they're cooked, the pepper skins should be slightly blistered and a little charred in places. Leave them until they're cool enough to handle, then tear them or leave them whole—whichever you prefer—and divide them among 4 plates. Drain the burrata, tear it, and serve it alongside the peppers and 'nduja. Serve some ciabatta on the side.

Roasted Veggies and Apple Salad

Prep time: 15 minutes | Cook time: 30 minutes | Serves 4

For the Salad:

¾ pound (340.2 g) young carrots (a mixture of colors is best, if you can find them)
3 tablespoons extra-virgin olive oil
Sea salt flakes and freshly ground black pepper, to taste
1¼ cups cooked Puy lentils
1 red Fresno chili and 1 green chili, halved, seeded, and very finely shredded
2 preserved lemons, rind only, finely shredded, plus 2 teaspoons brine from the jar
1 large or 2 medium tart apples
Juice of ½ lemon
Leaves from 10 mint sprigs, torn
¼ cup cilantro leaves

For the Dressing:

2 tablespoons white balsamic vinegar
$^1/_3$ cup extra-virgin olive oil (fruity rather than grassy)
1 fat garlic clove, finely grated
½-inch fresh ginger, peeled and finely grated
¼ teaspoon clear honey

1. Preheat the oven to 400ºF (205ºC).
2. Trim the carrots, but leave a bit of green tuft. If you can't find young carrots, halve or quarter larger ones lengthwise. Don't peel them, just wash them well. Place in a single layer in a bake pan. Add the olive oil, salt, and pepper, then toss to ensure the carrots are coated.
3. Bake in the oven for 30 to 35 minutes, or until tender. Be careful not to overcook them.
4. Make the dressing by putting the vinegar in a bowl and whisking in all the other ingredients with a fork. Season.
5. Put the lentils into a broad shallow serving bowl with half the chili and one-third of the preserved lemon. Season a little, then toss with about one- third of the dressing.
6. Halve and core the apple or apples (there's no need to peel them) and cut into matchsticks. Throw into a large mixing bowl with the lemon juice and add the carrots. Add the rest of the preserved lemons and chili, along with two-thirds of the herbs and the remaining dressing.
7. Throw the rest of the mint and cilantro into the lentils. Put the carrot and apple mixture on top, you should still be able to see the lentils around the sides and serve.

Black Bean and Tomato Salsa

Prep time: 10 minutes | Cook time: 0 minutes | Serves 4

1 garlic bud, roasted, peeled, and mashed
1 can black beans, drained and rinsed
½ cup finely chopped onion
1 cup finely chopped fresh tomato
2 tablespoons tomato paste
½ cup finely chopped green or red bell pepper
1 tablespoon finely chopped fresh
Cilantro
1 teaspoon chili powder
3 tablespoons lemon juice
Salt and freshly ground black pepper, to taste

1. Combine all the ingredients in a medium bowl, stirring well to blend, and adjust the seasonings to taste. Chill before serving.

CHAPTER 6 DESSERTS

Blueberry Pie Bars

Prep time: 10 minutes | Cook time: 25 minutes | Serves 9 bars

For the Graham Cracker Crust:

1½ cups graham cracker crumbs
6 tablespoons unsalted butter, melted
$^1/_3$ cup sugar

For the Filling:

2 large eggs
1 cup sugar
2 tablespoons all-purpose flour
Zest of 1 large lemon, divided (reserve some for garnish, optional)
Juice of 1 large lemon
¼ cup heavy (whipping) cream
2 cups fresh blueberries (reserve some for garnish, optional)

Make the Graham Cracker Crust

1. Select Convection Bake and preheat the oven to 325ºF (163ºC).
2. In a medium bowl, stir together the graham cracker crumbs, melted butter, and sugar until a sandy mixture forms. Press the mixture firmly into the bottom of an 8- or 9-inch square baking pan. Bake for 6 to 8 minutes.
3. Remove the crust from the oven, but leave the oven on.

Make the Filling

4. While the crust bakes, in a medium bowl, whisk the eggs and sugar until well combined.
5. Add the flour, lemon zest and juice, and heavy cream. Beat or whisk until well incorporated. Pour the filling over the prebaked crust, smoothing it into an even layer with a rubber spatula.
6. Sprinkle the blueberries over the top (they will begin to sink, which is fine!).
7. Lower the oven temperature to 300ºF (150ºC), and bake the bars for 18 to 22 minutes, until the edges just begin to brown and the center is firm.
8. Set the pan on a wire rack and cool to room temperature. Transfer the pan to the refrigerator and chill for at least 1 hour before serving. The bars will keep, covered, in the refrigerator for up to 3 days.
9. To serve, cut into squares and serve garnished with the reserved blueberries and grated lemon zest (if using).

Baked Shortbread Brown Sugar Bars

Prep time: 10 minutes | Cook time: 25 minutes | Makes 12 bars

For the Crust:

Nonstick baking spray, for preparing the baking dish
¼ cup confectioners' sugar
2 cups all-purpose flour
1 cup cold, unsalted butter, cut into small pieces

For the Filling:

8 tablespoons unsalted butter, melted
3 cups light brown sugar
4 large eggs
2 tablespoons white vinegar
1 tablespoon vanilla extract

Make the Crust

1. Select Convection Bake and preheat the oven to 325ºF (163ºC).
2. Line a 9-by-13-inch baking dish with parchment paper and spray it with baking spray.
3. In a large bowl, whisk the confectioners' sugar and flour.
4. Add the butter. Using your hands, a pastry cutter, two knives, or a mixing blade attachment on a mixer, cut it into the flour mixture until it is in small clumps. Press the flour mixture firmly into the prepared baking dish in an even layer. Bake for 7 to 9 minutes, until the crust is lightly brown and crisp.
5. Remove the crust from the oven and lower the oven temperature to 300ºF (150ºC).

Make the Filling

6. In a large bowl (use the same bowl you used for the crust), combine the melted butter and brown sugar and stir to combine.
7. Add the eggs, vinegar, and vanilla and whisk well to combine. Pour the filling over the prebaked crust and spread it into an even layer. Bake for 18 to 23 minutes, until the filling is set in the center. Transfer the pan to a wire rack and cool to room

temperature. Cover and refrigerate for at least 1 hour before serving. Serve chilled.

Apple Pie with Caramel Sauce

Prep time: 15 minutes | Cook time: 1 hour | Serves 8

For the Crust:

2½ cups all-purpose flour, plus more for the work surface
2 teaspoons sugar
1 teaspoon table salt
1 cup (2 sticks) cold, unsalted butter, cut into small pieces
4 to 6 tablespoons ice-cold water
1 large egg, for the egg wash
1 tablespoon water, for the egg wash
2 tablespoons coarse sugar, for sprinkling

For the Filling:

6 large apples, peeled, cored, and diced
½ cup sugar
2 teaspoons lemon zest
¼ cup freshly squeezed lemon juice
¼ cup all-purpose flour
1½ teaspoons ground cinnamon
1 cup caramel sauce, divided

Make the Crust

1. In a large bowl, stand mixer, or food processor, combine the flour, sugar, and salt and stir or pulse to mix.
2. Add the butter. Using your hands, a pastry cutter, two knives, or a mixing blade attachment on a mixer, cut it into the flour until the mixture begins to come together in crumbs.
3. While stirring or with the mixer or food processor running, slowly add the ice water, 1 tablespoon at a time, until the dough balls up and begins to pull away from the sides of the bowl. Remove the dough and form it into 2 equal-size disks. Wrap each disk in plastic wrap and refrigerate for about 20 minutes.

Make the Filling

4. While the dough chills, toss the apples with the sugar, lemon zest, lemon juice, flour, and cinnamon in a large bowl until well combined.

Assemble the Pie

5. On a lightly floured work surface, roll 1 dough ball into a 12-inch circle (⅛ inch thick). Place the dough in a 9-inch pie dish, pressing it gently into the bottom and sides. Trim off and discard any excess dough.
6. Spoon the apple mixture on top of the crust.
7. Pour ½ cup of caramel sauce over the apples.
8. Select Convection Bake and preheat the oven to 375ºF (190ºC).
9. On a lightly floured work surface, roll the remaining dough ball into a 12-inch circle about ⅛ inch thick. With a sharp knife, pizza cutter, or pastry cutter, cut 16 (½-inch-wide) strips. Weave the strips over the top of the pie in a crisscross lattice pattern and trim any excess from the edges. Crimp the dough around the edges to seal it and create a decorative edge.
10. In a small bowl, whisk the egg and water and brush the egg wash over the strips on top of the pie. Sprinkle the coarse sugar over the top.
11. Place the pie on a baking sheet and bake for about 20 minutes. Lower the oven temperature to 350ºF (180ºC) and bake for about 40 minutes more, until the filling is bubbling and the crust is golden brown and crisp.
12. Remove the pie from the oven and set on a wire rack to cool for at least 3 hours before serving. To serve, cut into wedges and drizzle some of the remaining ½ cup of caramel sauce over the top.

Golden Peach Upside-Down Cake

Prep time: 15 minutes | Cook time: 40 minutes | Serves

Butter, for preparing the baking pan

For the Topping:

½ cup light brown sugar
4 tablespoons unsalted butter, melted
5 peaches, peeled and sliced ¼ inch thick

For the Cake:

$1^1/_3$ cups all-purpose flour
1½ teaspoons baking powder
¼ teaspoon salt
8 tablespoons unsalted butter, at room temperature
$^1/_3$ cup sugar
$^1/_3$ cup light brown sugar
1 large egg

¼ cup milk
2 teaspoons vanilla extract
1. Select Convection Bake and preheat the oven to 325ºF (163ºC).
2. Butter the bottom and sides of a 9-inch round cake pan.

Make the Topping

3. In a small bowl, mix together the brown sugar and melted butter and spread it into the bottom of the prepared cake pan.
4. Starting from the middle of the pan, arrange the peach slices to cover the entire surface, layering the fruit as needed.

Make the Cake

5. In a small bowl, stir together the flour, baking powder, and salt.
6. In a medium bowl, using a handheld electric mixer, a stand mixer, or a wooden spoon, cream together the butter, sugar, and brown sugar.
7. Add the egg, milk, and vanilla and beat well to mix.
8. Add the dry ingredients and beat on low speed, or mix by hand, until fully incorporated. Spoon the batter evenly over the peaches and carefully smooth it into an even layer. Bake for 40 to 45 minutes, until golden brown and springy to the touch.
9. Remove the pan from the oven and let the cake cool in the pan for 5 minutes. To unmold the cake, run a sharp knife around the edge of the pan and place an inverted serving platter on top. Carefully invert the cake so it falls out onto the platter. Cut into wedges and serve.

Glazed Sweet Bundt Cake

Prep time: 10 minutes | Cook time: 55 minutes | Serves 8

For the Cake:

1½ cups unsalted butter, at room temperature, plus more for preparing the pan
2 cups light brown sugar
1 cup sugar
5 large eggs
3 cups all-purpose flour, plus more for preparing the pan
1 teaspoon table salt
1 cup sour cream, at room temperature
1 tablespoon vanilla extract

For the Glaze:

1 cup confectioners' sugar
2 tablespoons milk

Make the Cake

1. Select Convection Bake and preheat the oven to 300ºF (150ºC).
2. Butter and flour a 10-cup Bundt pan.
3. In a large bowl, using a wooden spoon or an electric mixer, cream together the butter, brown sugar, and sugar until the mixture is pale yellow and fluffy.
4. Add the eggs, one at a time, mixing after each addition until incorporated.
5. Add the flour, salt, sour cream, and vanilla and beat until just combined. Transfer the batter to the prepared pan and bake for 55 minutes to 1 hour.
6. Remove the cake from the oven and set on a wire rack to cool for 10 minutes before inverting it onto a cake platter and letting it cool completely.

Make the Glaze

7. In a small bowl, whisk the confectioners' sugar and milk until smooth. Drizzle the glaze over the completely cooled cake.

Marshmallow on Brownie

Prep time: 15 minutes | Cook time: 30 minutes | Serves 16 brownies

For the Graham Cracker Crust:

1½ cups graham cracker crumbs (about 10 full graham cracker sheets, crushed)
6 tablespoons unsalted butter, melted
$^{1}/_{3}$ cup sugar

For the Brownies:

8 tablespoons unsalted butter, at room temperature
7 ounces (198 g) semisweet or bittersweet chocolate, chopped
1 cup all-purpose flour
¼ teaspoon table salt
2 large eggs
½ cup sugar
½ cup light brown sugar
1 teaspoon vanilla extract

For the Topping:

36 marshmallows (use gelatin-free vegetarian marshmallows if that is a concern)

Make the Graham Cracker Crust

1. Select Convection Bake and preheat the oven to 325ºF (163ºC).
2. In a medium bowl, stir together the graham cracker crumbs, melted butter, and sugar until a sandy mixture forms. Press the mixture firmly into the bottom of an 8- or 9-inch square baking pan. Bake for 6 to 8 minutes. Remove the crust from the oven, but leave the oven on.

Make the Brownies

3. In a medium saucepan or double boiler over low heat, melt the butter and chocolate together, stirring continuously. Remove from the heat and let cool.
4. In a medium bowl, stir together the flour and salt.
5. In a large bowl, with a wooden spoon or an electric mixer, beat together the eggs, sugar, and brown sugar until pale and fluffy.
6. Stir in the vanilla and melted chocolate until incorporated.
7. Gently stir in the flour just until incorporated. Pour the chocolate batter over the crust. Bake for about 22 minutes. Remove the pan from the oven and turn the oven to broil.

Make the Topping

8. Cover the top of the brownies with a single layer of marshmallows standing on end. Broil for 1 to 2 minutes, just until the marshmallows are golden brown on top, watching carefully. Remove from the oven, cut into squares with a knife dipped in hot water, and serve warm.

Mexican Brownie Squares

Prep time: 10 minutes | Cook time: 25 minutes | Serves 8

½ cup unsalted butter, plus more for greasing
8 ounces (227 g) dark chocolate (60 to 72 percent cocoa)
1 cup sugar
2 teaspoons vanilla extract
Pinch salt
2 large eggs, at room temperature
1 teaspoon ground cinnamon
¼ teaspoon cayenne
¾ cup all-purpose flour

1. Select Convection Bake and preheat the oven to 350ºF (180ºC).
2. Line a 9-inch square baking pan with aluminum foil, with the ends extending over the edges of the pan on two sides. Butter the foil and pan.
3. In a small saucepan, gently melt the butter and chocolate together over low heat, stirring, just until melted. Remove from the heat and let cool slightly. Pour into a large bowl.
4. Stir in the sugar, vanilla, and salt. Add the eggs, one at a time, and stir until completely blended.
5. Mix the cinnamon and cayenne into the flour until evenly dispersed. Add the flour to the chocolate mixture and beat until incorporated, about a minute. The batter may be a bit grainy looking.
6. Pour the batter into the prepared pan and bake for 25 to 30 minutes, until a toothpick inserted into the center comes out with crumbs but no raw batter sticking to it. Let cool for about 10 minutes. Pick up the edges of the foil and carefully lift the brownies out of the pan. Peel off the foil and let cool for another 5 minutes. Cut into squares.

Easy Nutmeg Butter Cookies

Prep time: 10 minutes | Cook time: 11 minutes | Makes 4 dozen

½ cup (1 stick) unsalted butter, melted
1 cup sugar
1 teaspoon vanilla extract
¼ teaspoon kosher salt
1 large egg
1 cup all-purpose flour
1½ teaspoons freshly grated nutmeg

1. Select Convection Bake and preheat the oven to 350ºF (180ºC). Line two sheet pans with silicone baking mats (or use one sheet pan and bake in batches).
2. In a large bowl, mix together the butter and sugar. Stir in the vanilla and salt. Add the egg and beat until the mixture is smooth.
3. In a small bowl, whisk together the flour and nutmeg. Stir the flour mixture into the sugar and butter mixture just until blended.
4. Drop the batter by level teaspoons onto the prepared pans, leaving about 2 inches around the dough balls.
5. Bake for 11 to 12 minutes, or until the cookies have spread, the edges are golden brown, and the tops start to collapse. Let cool on the pans for

a few minutes, then transfer to a rack to cool completely.

Blueberry and Peach Crisp

Prep time: 15 minutes | Cook time: 30 minutes | Serves 4

For the Filling:

Nonstick cooking spray
5 ripe yellow peaches
1 cup fresh or frozen blueberries
1/3 cup granulated sugar
1 tablespoon all-purpose flour
1 teaspoon grated lemon zest

For the Topping:

½ cup quick-cooking oatmeal
1/3 cup brown sugar
1/3 cup all-purpose flour
¼ cup blanched slivered almonds
1 teaspoon ground cinnamon
½ teaspoon ground cardamom
Pinch salt
4 tablespoons unsalted butter or vegan margarine

1. To make the filling: Select Convection Bake and preheat the oven to 350ºF (180ºC). Spray a 9-inch square baking pan with cooking spray.
2. Peel and pit the peaches. Slice them about ½-inch thick, then cut the slices in half. You should have about 4 cups of slices. Put them in a medium bowl and add the blueberries, sugar, flour, and lemon zest. Toss gently. Pour into the prepared baking pan.
3. To make the topping: For the topping, mix together the oatmeal, brown sugar, flour, almonds, cinnamon, cardamom, and salt. With a pastry cutter or a large fork, cut in the butter until the mixture is crumbly. (Or use a food processor, but don't overprocess.)
4. Sprinkle the topping over the fruit. Bake for 30 minutes, or until the top is lightly browned and the peaches are bubbling. Let cool for about 15 minutes before cutting. Serve warm.

Chewy Bars

Prep time: 10 minutes | Cook time: 8 minutes | Serves 4

¾ cup peanut butter
½ cup (1 stick) unsalted butter, softened
½ cup packed brown sugar
½ cup granulated sugar
1 large egg
1 teaspoon vanilla extract
1½ cups all-purpose flour
½ teaspoon baking soda
1½ cups bittersweet chocolate chips, divided
¾ cup salted roasted peanuts, very coarsely chopped
1 cup caramel sauce

1. Select Convection Bake and preheat the oven to 350ºF (180ºC).
2. Beat the peanut butter, butter, and sugars in a stand mixer (or with a hand mixer) until creamy. Beat in the egg and vanilla.
3. In a small bowl, whisk together the flour and baking soda, then gradually beat the flour mixture into the peanut butter mixture. Stir in half the chocolate chips, distributing them evenly in the dough. Press into a 9-by-13-inch baking pan.
4. Sprinkle the remaining chocolate chips and the peanuts over the dough.
5. Bake for 8 minutes, or just until the top of the dough is set, then remove the pan from the oven, drizzle with the caramel, and return to the oven for 10 to 12 minutes, until the caramel is bubbling. Cool completely, then cut into bars.

Currant Carrot Cake with Icing

Prep time: 15 minutes | Cook time: 30 minutes | Serves 6

1 cup unbleached flour
1 teaspoon baking powder
1 teaspoon baking soda
½ cup evaporated skim milk
½ cup brown sugar
2 tablespoons vegetable oil
1 egg
1 cup grated carrots
½ cup chopped currants
¼ cup finely chopped pecans
Salt, to taste

For the Yogurt Cream Icing:

2 tablespoons plain yogurt
1 teaspoon vanilla extract
1 tablespoon reduced-fat cream cheese
1½ cups confectioners' sugar, sifted
Salt, to taste

1. Preheat the toaster oven to 350ºF (180ºC).
2. Combine all the ingredients in a medium bowl, stirring well to mix thoroughly.
3. Spread the batter in an oiled or nonstick 8½ × 8½ × 2-inch square baking (cake) pan.
4. Bake for 30 minutes, or until a toothpick inserted in the center comes out clean.
5. Meanwhile, stir together the icing ingredients in a small bowl, then beat with an electric mixer until smooth. Add more confectioners' sugar or yogurt until the icing is the consistency of very thick cream.
6. Cool the cake on a wire rack. Ice with yogurt cream icing.

Coconut Cake with Creamy Frosting

Prep time: 15 minutes | Cook time: 25 minutes | Serves 6

2 cups unbleached flour
2 teaspoons baking powder
1 cup skim or low-fat soy milk
2 tablespoons vegetable oil
1 teaspoon vanilla extract
1 egg, beaten
¾ cup sugar
Salt, to taste

For the Creamy Frosting:

1½ cups confectioners' sugar, sifted
3 tablespoons margarine
1 tablespoon fat-free half-and-half or skim milk
½ teaspoon vanilla extract
Salt, to taste
½ cup sweetened flaked coconut
1 (5-ounce / 142-g) can mandarin oranges, drained well

1. Preheat the toaster oven to 350ºF (180ºC).
2. Combine all the ingredients in a large bowl, mixing well.
3. Pour the cake batter into an oiled or nonstick 8½ × 8½ × 2-inch square baking (cake) pan.
4. Bake for 25 minutes, or until a toothpick inserted in the center comes out clean.
5. Combine all the ingredients except the flaked coconut and mandarin oranges (reserve for sprinkling and decorating later) in a medium bowl.
6. Beat with an electric mixer at high speed until light and fluffy. Add more confectioners' sugar if the frosting is too liquid or more fat-free half-and-half if the frosting is too stiff. It should be about the consistency of room-temperature peanut butter.
7. Ice with creamy frosting and sprinkle with coconut.

Tangy Orange-Glazed Brownies

Prep time: 10 minutes | Cook time: 40 minutes | Makes 12 squares

3 squares unsweetened chocolate
3 tablespoons margarine
1 cup sugar
½ cup orange juice
2 eggs
1½ cups unbleached flour
1 teaspoon baking powder
Salt, to taste
1 tablespoon grated orange zest

For the Orange Glaze:

1 cup orange juice
½ cup sugar

1. Broil the chocolate and margarine in an oiled or nonstick 8½ × 8½ × 2-inch square baking (cake) pan for 3 minutes, or until almost melted. Remove from the oven and stir until completely melted. Transfer the chocolate/margarine mixture to a medium bowl.
2. Beat in the sugar, orange juice, and eggs with an electric mixer. Stir in the flour, baking powder, salt, and orange zest and mix until well blended. Pour into the oiled or nonstick square cake pan.
3. Bake at 350ºF (180ºC). for 30 minutes, or until a toothpick inserted in the center comes out clean.
4. Combine the orange juice and sugar in a small bowl and mix well. Transfer the mixture to a baking pan.
5. Broil for 10 minutes, stirring after 5 minutes, or until the sugar is dissolved and the liquid is reduced. Drizzle on top of brownies and cool. Cut into squares and serve with scoops of vanilla frozen yogurt or orange sherbet.

6. Make holes over the entire top by piercing with a fork or toothpick. Paint with orange glaze and cut into squares.

Spice Cake with Creamy Frosting

Prep time: 20 minutes | Cook time: 25 minutes | Serves 6

1 cup applesauce
¼ cup skim milk or low-fat soy milk
1 tablespoon vegetable oil
½ cup brown sugar
1 egg
1½ cups unbleached flour
1 teaspoon baking powder
½ teaspoon baking soda
¼ teaspoon grated nutmeg
½ teaspoon ground cinnamon
½ teaspoon grated orange zest
Salt, to taste

For the Creamy Frosting:

1½ cups confectioners' sugar, sifted
3 tablespoons margarine
1 tablespoon fat-free half-and-half or skim milk
½ teaspoon vanilla extract
Salt, to taste
½ cup sweetened flaked coconut
1 (5-ounce / 142-g) can mandarin oranges, drained well

1. Preheat the toaster oven to 350ºF (180ºC).
2. Stir together the applesauce, milk, oil, sugar, and egg in a small bowl. Set aside.
3. Combine the flour, baking powder, nutmeg, cinnamon, orange zest, and salt in a medium bowl. Add the applesauce mixture and stir to mix well. Pour the batter into an oiled or nonstick 8½ × 8½ × 2-inch square baking (cake) pan.
4. Bake for 25 minutes, or until a toothpick inserted in the center comes out clean. Frost with creamy frosting.

Lemon Torte with Cream Cheese Frosting

Prep time: 10 minutes | Cook time: 8 minutes | Serves 6

First Mixture:

¼ cup margarine, at room temperature
½ teaspoon grated lemon zest
3 egg yolks
¼ cup sugar
$^{1}/_{3}$ cup unbleached flour
3 tablespoons cornstarch

Second Mixture:

3 egg whites
2 tablespoons sugar

For the Cream Cheese Frosting:

1 cup confectioners' sugar
1 tablespoon fat-free half-and-half
2 tablespoons reduced-fat cream cheese
1 teaspoon lemon juice

1. Beat together the first mixture ingredients in a medium bowl with an electric mixer until the mixture is smooth. Set aside. Clean the electric mixer beaters.
2. Beat the second mixture together: Beat the egg whites into soft peaks in a medium bowl, gradually adding the sugar, and continue beating until the peaks are stiff. Fold the first mixture into the second mixture to make the torte batter.
3. Pour ½ cup torte batter into a small oiled or nonstick 3½ × 7½ × 2¼-inch loaf pan.
4. Broil for 1 or 2 minutes, or until lightly browned. Remove from the oven.
5. Pour and spread evenly another ½ cup batter on top of the first layer. Broil again for 1 or 2 minutes, or until lightly browned. Repeat the process until all the batter is used up.
6. Beat the frosting ingredients in a medium bowl with an electric mixer until light and fluffy, adding more confectioners' sugar if the mixture is too liquid or more cream cheese if the mixture is too stiff. It should have the consistency of room-temperature peanut butter.
7. When cool, run a knife around the sides to loosen and invert onto a plate. Chill. Frost with cream cheese frosting and serve chilled.

Glazed Chocolate Cake

Prep time: 15 minutes | Cook time: 40 minutes | Serves 10

For the Cake:

7 ounces (198 g) unsalted butter, at room temperature, plus more for the pan
5½ ounces (155.9 g) 70% cocoa solids dark chocolate, broken into pieces
1½ cups dark brown sugar
4 extra-large eggs, at room temperature, lightly beaten
3 tablespoons cocoa powder
1¾ cups all-purpose flour
1 teaspoon baking powder
Pinch of fine sea salt
½ cup full-bodied red wine (Merlot is perfect here)
Finely grated zest of 1 orange

For the Glaze:

4½ ounces 70% cocoa solids dark chocolate, broken into pieces
½ cup heavy cream
2 tablespoons port
3 tablespoons confectioners' sugar, sifted

1. Preheat the oven to 350ºF (180ºC). Butter a 9-in spring form cake pan and line the bottom with parchment paper.
2. Put the chocolate in a heatproof bowl set over a pan of gently simmering water (the bottom of the bowl shouldn't touch the water). Melt the chocolate, stirring a little to help it along. Remove the bowl and leave it to cool a little.
3. Cream the butter and sugar with electric beaters until lighter in color and fluffy. Gradually add the eggs, beating well after each addition.
4. In a bowl, sift together the cocoa, flour, baking powder, and salt, then fold the mixture into the batter. Stir in the red wine and the orange zest, then the melted chocolate. Scrape into the prepared pan and bake for 40 minutes, or until a skewer inserted into the middle comes out clean. Allow the cake to cool in the pan, then turn it out onto a wire rack to cool completely.
5. For the glaze, put the chocolate into a heatproof bowl and melt as before. Stir in the cream with the port until the mixture is smooth, then whisk in the confectioners' sugar. Leave this to cool a little (though don't leave it until it has set), then pour it over the cake. Let the glaze set a bit before serving.
6. A glass of red dessert wine (look for Maury from France, or the Greek sweet red wine Mavrodaphne) is lovely with this.

Rice Pudding with Quince Jelly and Blackberry

Prep time: 10 minutes | Cook time: 40 minutes | Serves 4 to 6

For the Rice Pudding:

3½ tablespoons unsalted butter, plus more for the dish
3 tablespoons superfine sugar
Scant ½ cup short-grain rice (not risotto rice)
1 quart whole milk
$^{2}/_{3}$ cup heavy cream
Pinch of salt
Lots of freshly grated nutmeg
Finely grated zest of ½ unwaxed lemon
¼ teaspoon vanilla extract

To Serve

Quince jelly (blackcurrant jelly is a good substitute)
$^{1}/_{3}$ pound (151.2 g) blackberries

1. Preheat the oven to 325ºF (163ºC) and butter a 2-quart baking dish.
2. Put the butter, sugar, rice, milk, and cream into a saucepan and bring gently to a boil, stirring to help the sugar dissolve. Add the salt, nutmeg, lemon zest, and vanilla extract and return to a simmer.
3. Simmer for about 4 minutes, stirring all the time, until you can feel that the rice grains have become slightly (only slightly) swollen. Pour the mixture into the prepared dish and bake for 2 hours. By this time the rice should be creamy and cooked, but shouldn't be dry or overly sticky.
4. As the pudding looks beautiful baked—it develops a lovely golden skin on top—take it to the table in the baking dish, and put the quince jelly and the blackberries in separate serving bowls so people can help themselves.

Rum-Plums with Brown Sugar Cream

Prep time: 10 minutes | Cook time: 15 minutes | Serves 6

For the Cream:

¾ cup plus 2 tablespoons heavy cream
$^{2}/_{3}$ cup Greek yogurt
3 to 4 heaping tablespoons dark brown sugar

For the Plums:

1¾ pounds (793.8 g) plums (preferably crimson-fleshed), halved and pitted

2 slices of crystallized ginger, very finely chopped

½ cup light brown sugar

½ teaspoon ground ginger

3 broad strips of lime zest, plus juice of 1 lime

$^{2}/_{3}$ cup dark rum, plus 3 tablespoons

1. Make the cream about 12 hours before you want to serve it. Lightly whip the heavy cream, then fold in the yogurt. Put this in a bowl and sprinkle evenly with the sugar. Cover with plastic wrap and refrigerate. The sugar will become soft and molasses-like.
2. Preheat the oven to 375ºF (190ºC).
3. Put the plums into a bake pan or a big ovenproof dish or gratin dish in which they can lie in a single layer (snugly; you don't want the juices around them to reduce and burn). Arrange the fruits so they are cut sides up. Scatter the crystallized ginger around the plums. Mix the sugar with the ground ginger and sprinkle it over the top. Squeeze the lime juice over and tuck the pieces of lime zest under the fruits, then pour the $^{2}/_{3}$ cup rum around them.
4. Bake for 15 to 30 minutes (how long it takes depends on the ripeness of the plums). The fruit should be tender when pierced with a sharp knife, but not collapsing. Leave to cool completely; the juices should thicken as they cool. If they aren't thick enough, drain off the juices and boil them in a saucepan until they become more syrupy. Add the remaining 3 tablespoons of rum. Serve the plums, at room temperature, with the brown sugar cream.

Roasted Stone Fruit

Prep time: 10 minutes | Cook time: 30 minutes | Serves 8

2 pounds (907 g) stone fruit, a mixture of peaches, nectarines, plums, and apricots is good here

2 tablespoons superfine sugar

Finely grated zest of 1 unwaxed lemon, plus juice of ½ lemon

2½ ounces (70.9 g) good-quality marzipan

½ tablespoon orange flower water

$^{1}/_{3}$ cup all-purpose flour

¼ cup almond flour

4 tablespoons cold unsalted butter, cut into cubes

2 tablespoons sliced almonds

Confectioners' sugar, to dust (optional)

Whipped cream or crème fraîche, to serve

1. Preheat the oven to 400ºF (205ºC).
2. Halve and pit all the fruit. Cut the larger fruits (like peaches and nectarines) into 6 wedges (each half into 3). Put all the fruit into a dish, sprinkle it with the sugar, lemon zest, and lemon juice, and turn it over with your hands. Take 1 ounce of the marzipan and put little nuggets of this in among the fruit. Break the rest of the marzipan into little balls, but reserve it for now. Sprinkle the orange flower water over the fruit.
3. Put the flour, almond flour, and butter into a bowl and rub them together with your fingertips. You want to end up with a mixture that looks like small pebbles and gravel. Sprinkle this over the top of the fruit, then put the balls of marzipan on top, too, leaving patches of the fruit completely uncovered. Bake for 30 minutes, or until the fruit is completely tender and the crumbs are golden, scattering over the sliced almonds halfway through the cooking time.
4. Leave to cool a bit (I like it at room temperature, but you might prefer it warm) and dust a little confectioners' sugar over the top, if you want.
5. Serve with whipped cream or crème fraîche.

Rhubarb with Sloe Gin and Rosemary

Prep time: 10 minutes | Cook time: 30 minutes | Serves 44

1½ pounds (680.4 g) hothouse or main crop rhubarb stalks, all about the same thickness

½ cup granulated sugar

Finely grated zest of ½ orange

7 tablespoons sloe gin

3 tablespoons orange juice

2 rosemary sprigs, bruised

Whipped cream or heavy cream, to serve

1. Preheat the oven to 350ºF (180ºC).
2. Remove any leaves from the rhubarb and trim the bottoms. Cut into 1¼in lengths and put them into a large ovenproof dish. Scatter the sugar and zest on top and turn it all over with your hands, then pour in the sloe gin, orange juice, and 2 tablespoons

of water, and finally tuck the rosemary sprigs under the rhubarb.

3. Cover tightly with foil, then bake for 30 minutes or so (the time this takes will depend on the thickness of the stalks, start checking after 20 minutes by piercing them with a sharp knife). The rhubarb should be tender, but holding its shape and not collapsing.

4. Remove from the oven and leave to cool a bit in the dish. Eat warm, at room temperature, or chilled, with whipped cream or heavy cream.

Apricot Brioche with Croûtes Fraîche

Prep time: 10 minutes | Cook time: 25 minutes | Serves 6

6 thick slices of brioche
2 tablespoons superfine sugar, plus 4 teaspoons
¼ cup amaretto or Marsala
5 tablespoons very soft unsalted butter
3¾ ounces (106.3 g) good-quality marzipan, broken into small chunks
12 small ripe apricots, or 6 plums, pitted and quartered
Juice of ½ lemon
Generous ¼ cup sliced almonds (optional)
Confectioners' sugar, to dust (optional)
Crème fraîche, to serve

1. Preheat the oven to 400ºF (205ºC).
2. Put the brioche slices on a sheet pan or in a bake pan in which they can lie in a single layer.
3. Spoon the 2 tablespoons sugar into a small heatproof bowl and pour in ¼ cup of boiling water. Stir until dissolved, then leave this simple syrup to cool. Stir in the amaretto or Marsala.
4. Spoon the cooled syrup over the brioche slices, covering both sides.
5. Carefully, because the brioche will be very soft now, butter each slice on both sides.
6. Arrange chunks of marzipan on top, then add the apricot quarters. Squeeze on the lemon juice and sprinkle with the 4 teaspoons of superfine sugar.
7. Bake for 25 minutes, sprinkling on the almonds, if using, after 15 minutes. The apricots should be tender and the bread and marzipan both golden.
8. Leave to cool a little (the slices will be very hot), then sift over some confectioners' sugar, if you want. Serve with crème fraîche.

Sour Cherry Brioche Pudding

Prep time: 10 minutes | Cook time: 45 minutes | Serves 8

1 cup dried sour cherries
Scant ½ cup unsweetened pomegranate juice
1¼ cups heavy cream
1¼ cups whole milk
Pinch of sea salt
Seeds from 2 cardamom pods, ground
3 extra-large eggs, plus 1 extra-large egg yolk
generous ½ cup superfine sugar
9 ounces (255 g) brioche loaf
2½ tablespoons unsalted butter, softened
1 teaspoon rose water, or to taste
Squeeze of lemon or lime juice
Confectioners' sugar, to dust

1. Put the dried cherries in a small saucepan and add enough pomegranate juice to just cover. Bring to a boil, then take off the heat and leave the cherries to sit and plump up (they need at least 30 minutes, but longer is fine).
2. Bring the cream, milk, and salt to a boil in a heavy-bottomed saucepan with the cardamom, then leave for 15 minutes off the heat. Beat the eggs, egg yolk, and sugar together. Pour the warm milk mixture onto this, stirring constantly.
3. Slice the brioche, butter it, and layer it in a 2 quart ovenproof dish, scattering the soaked cherries and any leftover pomegranate juice on as you layer the bread (try to get most of the cherries under the bread, or they might burn). Add some rose water to the egg and cream mixture—not too much—and a squeeze of lemon or lime juice, then taste it. You should be able to detect the rose water, but it shouldn't be too strong. Brands differ in strength, so you have to taste and decide if you need a little more.
4. Pour the egg and milk mixture evenly over the layers of bread. Leave the pudding to sit for 30 minutes; this will make it lighter.
5. Preheat the oven to 375ºF (190ºC).
6. Put the dish into a bake pan and carefully pour enough boiling water into the pan to come about one-third of the way up the sides of the dish.

Bake for 40 to 45 minutes, or until puffy, golden, and just set on the top. Remove the dish from the roasting tin and leave to cool slightly—the pudding will continue to cook in the residual heat for a while—then dust with confectioners' sugar before serving.

Cassis and Bay Baked Pears with Blackberry

Prep time: 5 minutes | Cook time: 35 minutes | Serves 6

6 just-ripe pears
½ cup cassis
1¼ cups red wine
¼ cup superfine sugar
3 bay leaves
5½ ounces (155.9 g) blackberries

1. Preheat the oven to 375ºF (190ºC).
2. Halve the pears, you don't need to peel or core them, and put them, cut sides up, into a gratin dish in which the fruit can sit quite snugly in a single layer. Pour the cassis and red wine over the pears, sprinkle with the sugar, and tuck the bay leaves under the fruit.
3. Begin to bake. Spoon the juices over the pears from time to time—until the fruits are tender right through to the center (how long this takes depends on the ripeness of the fruit, start checking after 20 minutes, but it could take as long as 35 minutes). It's a good idea to turn the pears over a couple of times while they're cooking.
4. By the time the fruit is cooked, the juice around it won't be thick, but should be syrupy and sweet enough to serve as it is. If you don't think it is, then remove the pears and bay leaves and reduce the juices by boiling them for a little while, leave to cool, then pour them back into the dish with the pears.
5. Add the berries about 30 minutes before you want to serve, spooning the juices over them, otherwise they get very soft sitting in the red wine syrup.

Passion Fruit, Lime, and Coconut Pudding

Prep time: 10 minutes | Cook time: 45 minutes | Serves 4 to 6

9 tablespoons unsalted butter, at room temperature, plus more for the dish
$1^{2}/_{3}$ cups superfine sugar
4 extra-large eggs, separated
½ cup all-purpose flour
¾ teaspoon baking powder
⅛ teaspoon salt
½ cup dried shredded coconut
1¾ cups whole milk
Finely grated zest and juice of 3 limes
5 large, juicy passion fruits, or 6 smaller fruits
Confectioners' sugar, to serve
Whipped cream, to serve

1. Preheat the oven to 350ºF (180ºC). Butter a 2-quart ovenproof dish.
2. Throw the butter and sugar into a food processor and process until light and fluffy. Add the egg yolks and whizz the mixture, then add the flour, baking powder, salt, and coconut, alternating with the milk, blending just until you have a smooth batter. Add the lime zest and juice, then scrape the batter into a large bowl.
3. Halve the passion fruits and scoop the pulp and seeds into a sieve placed over the bowl of batter. Push the pulp through the sieve into the batter, then add two-thirds of the black seeds, too (discard the remaining seeds).
4. Beat the egg whites until stiff. Using a large metal spoon, fold one-third of them into the batter to lighten it, then fold in the rest. Spoon into the prepared dish and set it in a bake pan. Pour enough boiling water into the bake pan to come halfway up the sides of the baking dish and bake for 45 minutes.
5. Allow the pudding to cool a little when it comes out of the oven, then sift confectioners' sugar over the top and serve with lightly whipped cream.

Nectarines with Pistachio Topping

Prep time: 10 minutes | Cook time: 30 minutes | Serves 6

6 nectarines, halved and pitted
$^{2}/_{3}$ cup shelled unsalted pistachios
Finely grated zest of ½ unwaxed lemon
1½ tablespoons superfine sugar
1 medium egg, lightly beaten

3 teaspoons rose water
1¼ cups apple juice
Confectioners' sugar, to dust
Nougat, to serve (optional)
Heavy cream, to serve

1. Preheat the oven to 375ºF (190ºC).
2. Put the nectarine halves in a gratin dish in which they can lie in a single layer without too much space around them (otherwise the apple juice will reduce and burn).
3. Crush the pistachios roughly using a mortar and pestle, then mix in the lemon zest, sugar, egg, and 1 teaspoon of the rose water. Fill the cavity of each nectarine with this stuffing, mounding it over the top if you have too much.
4. Mix the apple juice with the rest of the rose water and pour it around the nectarines. Bake for 30 to 45 minutes (the time it takes depends on the ripeness of the fruit). The nectarines should be tender and slightly caramelized on top.
5. Serve the fruit at room temperature, with a little confectioners' sugar sifted on top and some of the cooking juices spooned around, and pieces of nougat, if you like. Cream never goes amiss, of course.

Mincemeat and Cranberry Stuffed Apple

Prep time: 15 minutes | Cook time: 50 minutes | Serves 8

For the Apples and Toasted Rye:

1 tablespoon unsalted butter
1 cup coarse rye or pumpernickel breadcrumbs
Packed ¼ cup light brown sugar
8 tart apples
8 ounces (227 g) mincemeat
½ cup dried cranberries
Finely grated zest of ½ orange
2 tablespoons roughly chopped walnuts or hazelnuts
$1^2/_3$ cups dry hard cider, plus more if needed

For the Cream:

1¼ cups heavy cream
2½ tablespoons light brown sugar, or to taste
3 tablespoons apple brandy or Calvados

1. Preheat the oven to 375ºF (190ºC).
2. For the rye crumbs, melt the butter in a frying pan, then cook until it starts to brown a little. Remove from the heat and stir in the breadcrumbs and sugar. Spread this out on a baking sheet (it's important that the mixture is not in clumps) and bake for 20 minutes, tossing a few times during baking, until toasted. Let cool.
3. Slice the top off each apple to make a lid about 2in across, then core each one. Remove a little of the flesh around the core, too (don't throw it away, use it for a smoothie or something).
4. Put the apples in an ovenproof dish or bake pan in which they can sit close to each other; you don't want masses of space around them.
5. Mix the mincemeat with the cranberries, orange zest, and nuts. Spoon this into each apple, sprinkling any leftovers into the dish, then put the apple lids on. Pour the cider around the apples.
6. Bake for 30 to 40 minutes, or until the apples are completely tender, spooning the juices up over them every so often. Do keep an eye on the apples, as they can go from tender to burst and falling apart very suddenly.
7. Whip the cream until it's holding its shape, then whisk in the brown sugar and apple brandy or Calvados. Serve the apples with their juices, adding a dollop of the apple brandy cream and a scattering of the rye crumbs.

Thin Crepes

Prep time: 5 minutes | Cook time: 4 minutes | Serves 6

½ cup unbleached flour
¾ cup skim milk
1 egg
2 teaspoons vegetable oil
Salt, to taste

1. Whisk together all the ingredients in a small bowl until smooth. Set aside.
2. Preheat an oiled or nonstick 9¾-inch round pie pan by placing it under the broiler for 2 minutes, or until the pan is heated but not smoking. Remove from the oven and spoon 2 tablespoons crepe batter into the pan, tilting the pan to spread the batter evenly into a circle. Return to the broiler.
3. Broil for 4 minutes, or until the crepe is cooked but not browned. Remove the pan from the oven and invert onto paper towels to cool and drain. Repeat the procedure with the remaining batter.

Onion-Buttermilk Cheese Biscuits

Prep time: 10 minutes | Cook time: 15 minutes | Serves 4

2 cups unbleached flour
3 tablespoons margarine, at room temperature
¾ cup low-fat buttermilk
4 teaspoons baking powder
1 teaspoon garlic powder
¼ cup grated Parmesan cheese
3 tablespoons finely chopped onion
2 tablespoons chopped fresh parsley
Salt, to taste

1. Preheat the toaster oven to 400ºF (205ºC).
2. Blend all the ingredients in a medium bowl with a fork, then press together to form a dough ball.
3. Knead the dough on a lightly floured surface just until smooth.
4. Roll the dough to ½-inch thickness and cut with a round 3-inch cookie cutter. Place on an oiled or nonstick 6½ × 10-inch baking sheet or in an oiled or nonstick 8½ × 8½ × 2-inch square baking (cake) pan.
5. Bake for 15 minutes, or until lightly browned.

CHAPTER 7 BREADS

Buttery Yeast-Raised Pan Rolls

Prep time: 10 minutes | Cook time: 13 minutes | Makes 15 rolls

2 (¼-ounce / 7.1-g) packets active dry yeast
½ cup warm water
4½ cups all-purpose flour
2 tablespoons sugar
1½ teaspoons kosher salt
1 large egg, beaten
1 cup warm milk
¾ cup unsalted butter, melted, divided

1. In a large bowl, dissolve the yeast in the warm water and let stand until bubbly, about 15 minutes.
2. Add about half the flour, the sugar, and salt and stir until well combined. Add the egg, warm milk, and 6 tablespoons of melted butter. Beat for a few minutes until thoroughly combined. Stir in the remaining flour.
3. Cover the bowl with plastic wrap or a clean towel, and let rise in a warm place until doubled in volume, about 45 minutes.
4. Pour 3 tablespoons of the remaining melted butter in a 9-by-13-inch baking pan and tilt the pan to spread it evenly. Briefly beat down the batter and spoon it out into 15 fairly even scoops in the pan. Cover lightly and let rise until almost doubled, about 30 minutes.
5. Select Convection Bake and preheat the oven to 400ºF (205ºC).
6. Drizzle the remaining 3 tablespoons of melted butter over the rolls. Bake for 13 to 15 minutes, until golden brown and puffed. Let cool for a few minutes and serve warm.

Multigrain Sesame Sandwich Bread

Prep time: 10 minutes | Cook time: 50 minutes | Makes 1 loaf

¾ cup rolled oats
2 tablespoons finely ground bulgur wheat
2 tablespoons unsalted butter
3 tablespoons brown sugar
2 teaspoons kosher salt
1 cup boiling water
2 (¼-ounce / 7.1-g) packets active dry yeast
¾ cup warm milk
¼ cup toasted sesame seeds
2 cups all-purpose flour
1 cup whole-wheat flour

1. In a large bowl, combine the oatmeal, bulgur wheat, butter, brown sugar, and salt. Pour the boiling water over the mixture and stir to combine. Let cool to room temperature, stirring occasionally.
2. In a small bowl, dissolve the yeast in the warm milk. After a few minutes, when it's starting to bubble, pour it into the grain mixture. Add the sesame seeds and both flours and stir to combine.
3. Knead the dough on a floured board for about 10 minutes. The dough will be soft but should not be sticky.
4. Place in an oiled bowl and cover the bowl with plastic wrap or a clean towel. Let rise in a warm place until doubled in size, about 40 minutes.
5. Oil a 9-by-5-inch loaf pan. Punch the dough down and pat out into an 8-by-10-inch rectangle. Starting with a short side, pull the sides into the center to form a loaf shape. Place the dough in the prepared pan, seam-side down. Cover with plastic wrap and let rise for 20 minutes, but no longer.
6. Select Convection Bake and preheat the oven to 350ºF (180ºC).
7. Bake the loaf for 50 to 55 minutes, until the top is browned and the bread sounds hollow when tapped. Let cool for 5 minutes, then remove from the pan and cool completely on a rack.

Italian Flatbread Flavored with Olive Oil

Prep time: 10 minutes | Cook time: 20 minutes | Serves 6 to 8

2 teaspoons sugar
2 cups warm water
1 (¼-ounce / 7.1-g) packet active dry yeast
4½ cups all-purpose flour, plus more for kneading
2 teaspoons kosher salt

4 tablespoons extra-virgin olive oil, divided, plus more for dipping (optional)
1 cup black or green pitted olives (such as kalamata or Greek), very coarsely chopped
1 tablespoon fresh thyme leaves
1. In a large bowl, stir the sugar into the warm water. Sprinkle in the yeast, and stir with a fork. Let stand until the yeast dissolves, about 10 minutes.
2. Add the flour, salt, and 1 tablespoon of oil and stir to blend well (the dough will be sticky). Knead the dough on a floured surface, adding more flour as necessary, until smooth and elastic, about 10 minutes. Form the dough into a ball. Oil a large bowl and add the dough, turning to coat. Cover the bowl with plastic wrap or a warm towel and let rise in a warm area until doubled, about 1 hour.
3. Punch down the dough; knead into a ball again, and return to the same bowl. Cover with plastic wrap and let rise until doubled, about 45 minutes.
4. Coat a sheet pan with 1 tablespoon of the oil. Punch down the dough and transfer it to the pan. Press the dough out into a rectangle that fills the pan. Using your fingertips, make even indentations all over the dough. Drizzle the remaining 2 tablespoons of oil over the dough. Sprinkle evenly with the olives and thyme. Let the dough rise, uncovered, until puffy, about 25 minutes.
5. Select Convection Bake and preheat the oven to 475ºF (245ºC). Bake the focaccia until brown and crusty, about 20 minutes. Serve warm or at room temperature, with additional oil for dipping, if desired.

Rosemary Bread Loaf

Prep time: 10 minutes | Cook time: 15 minutes | Serves 6

3 tablespoons olive oil
2 tablespoons margarine
1 teaspoon garlic
2 tablespoons grated Parmesan cheese
1 tablespoon finely chopped fresh rosemary leaves
½ teaspoon freshly ground black pepper
Salt, to taste
1 French baguette, sliced 2 inches thick
1. Preheat the toaster oven to 350ºF (180ºC).
2. Combine the all the ingredients except the French baguette in a small bowl, blending well with a fork. Adjust the seasonings to taste.
3. Spread the mixture on both sides of the bread slices and wrap the loaf in aluminum foil.
4. Bake for 10 minutes. Remove from the oven and peel back the foil, exposing the top of the bread loaf. Bake for another 5 minutes, or until the top is lightly browned.

Classic Popovers

Prep time: 5 minutes | Cook time: 30 minutes | Makes 6 to 9 popovers

2 eggs
1 cup skim milk
2 tablespoons vegetable oil
1 cup unbleached flour
Salt, to taste
1. Preheat the toaster oven to 400ºF (205ºC).
2. Beat all the ingredients in a medium bowl with an electric mixer at high speed until smooth. The batter should be the consistency of heavy cream.
3. Fill the pans of a 6-muffin tin three-quarters full.
4. Bake for 20 minutes, then reduce the heat to 350ºF (180ºC). and bake for 10 minutes, or until golden brown.

Ritzy Stuffed Bread

Prep time: 15 minutes | Cook time: 40 minutes | Makes 1 loaf

First Mixture:
1 apple, peeled and grated
1 carrot, peeled and grated
1 cup unbleached flour
2 teaspoons baking powder
$^{1}/_{3}$ cup chopped walnuts
$^{1}/_{3}$ cup raisins
$^{1}/_{3}$ cup rolled oats
$^{1}/_{3}$ cup shredded sweetened coconut
Blending Mixture:
1 banana
1 egg
1 cup low-fat buttermilk
2 tablespoons dark brown sugar
2 tablespoons vegetable oil
Salt, to taste
1. Preheat the toaster oven to 375ºF (190ºC).

2. Combine all the first mixture ingredients in a medium bowl and stir to mix well. Set aside.
3. Process all the blending mixture ingredients in a blender or food processor until the mixture is smooth. Add to the first mixture ingredients and stir to mix thoroughly. Transfer to an oiled or nonstick 8½ × 4½ × 2¼-inch regular size loaf pan.
4. Bake for 40 minutes, or until a toothpick inserted in the center comes out clean and the top is well browned.

Fruity Raisin and Almond Bread

Prep time: 10 minutes | Cook time: 35 minutes | Serves 6

2 cups unbleached flour
3 tablespoons margarine
4¾ cup low-fat buttermilk
5 teaspoons baking powder
1 egg, beaten
2 tablespoons honey
¼ cup chopped raisins
½ cup chopped dried fruit
3 tablespoons chopped almonds
4½ teaspoon grated nutmeg
Salt, to taste

1. Preheat the toaster oven to 400ºF (205ºC).
2. Combine all the ingredients in a large bowl, stirring well. Pour the batter into an oiled or nonstick regular-size 8½ × 4½ × $^2/_3$-inch loaf pan or 2 small-size 3½ × 7½ × 2¼-inch loaf pans.
3. Bake for 35 minutes, or until a toothpick inserted in the center comes out clean.

Plain Yogurt Bread

Prep time: 10 minutes | Cook time: 40 minutes | Makes 1 loaf

3 cups unbleached flour
4 teaspoons baking powder
2 teaspoons sugar
Salt, to taste
1 cup plain nonfat yogurt
¼ cup vegetable oil
1 egg, eaten, to brush the top

1. Preheat the toaster oven to 375ºF (190ºC).
2. Combine the flour, baking powder, sugar, and salt in a large bowl. Make a hole in the center and spoon in the yogurt and oil.
3. Stir the flour into the center. When the dough is well mixed, turn it out onto a lightly floured surface and knead for 8 minutes, until the dough is smooth and elastic. Place the dough in an oiled or nonstick regular-size 8½ × 4½ × 2¼-inch loaf pan. Brush the top with the beaten egg.
4. Bake for 40 minutes, or until a toothpick inserted in the center comes out clean and the loaf is browned. Invert on a wire rack to cool.

Country Yeast-Raised Bread

Prep time: 10 minutes | Cook time: 30 minutes | Makes 1 loaf

Yeast Mixture:

1(¼-ounce / 7.1-g) package active dry yeast
¼ cup skim milk, at room temperature
1 teaspoon brown sugar

Flour Mixture:

¾ cup tepid water
2½ cups unbleached flour
1 egg
2 teaspoons granulated sugar
2 tablespoons vegetable oil
2 tablespoons wheat germ
Salt, to taste
Vegetable oil
1 egg, beaten, to brush the top

1. Combine the yeast mixture ingredients in a large bowl and let stand for 10 minutes, or until the yeast is dissolved and foamy.
2. Add the flour mixture ingredients to the yeast mixture, blending well. Turn out the mixture on a lightly floured surface.
3. Knead the dough for 6 minutes, or until smooth and elastic. Return the dough to the large bowl, cover with a clean damp towel, and put in a warm place for 1 hour, or until doubled in size.
4. Punch down the dough and turn out onto a lightly floured surface. Knead for 2 minutes, then place the dough in an oiled or nonstick regular size 8½ × 4½ × 2¼-inch loaf pan. Brush the loaf with vegetable oil, cover the pan with a damp towel, and place in a warm place for 1 hour, or until doubled in size. Brush the loaf with the beaten egg.
5. Preheat the toaster oven to 375ºF (190ºC).

6. Bake for 30 minutes, or until a toothpick inserted in the middle comes out clean and the top is browned. Sharply tap the pan to loosen the loaf, invert, and place on a rack to cool.

Corn Breakfast Bread

Prep time: 10 minutes | Cook time: 20 minutes | Serves 6

1 cup cornmeal
¾ cup unbleached flour
2 tablespoons sugar
4 teaspoons baking powder
1 egg, beaten
1 cup skim milk
2 tablespoons vegetable oil
Salt, to taste

1. Preheat the toaster oven to 425ºF (220ºC).
2. Combine all the ingredients in a medium bowl and mix just to blend. The batter will be slightly lumpy. Pour into an oiled or nonstick regular-size 8½ × 4½ × 2¼-inch loaf pan.
3. Bake for 20 minutes, or until a toothpick inserted in the center comes out clean.

Zucchini Cheese Bread

Prep time: 10 minutes | Cook time: 30 minutes | Serves 6

1 cup grated zucchini
2 tablespoons grated onion
2 tablespoons grated Parmesan Cheese
½ cup skim milk
1 egg
2 tablespoons vegetable oil
1½ cups unbleached flour
1 tablespoon baking powder
Salt, to taste

1. Preheat the toaster oven to 375ºF (190ºC).
2. Stir together all the ingredients in a medium bowl until smooth. Pour the batter into an oiled or nonstick regular-size 8½ × 4½ × 2¼-inch loaf pan.
3. Bake for 30 minutes, or until a toothpick inserted in the center comes out clean.

Basil and Pine Nuts Bread

Prep time: 10 minutes | Cook time: 17 minutes | Serves 6

3 tablespoons olive oil
2 garlic cloves
¼ cup pine nuts (pignoli)
½ cup fresh basil leaves
2 plum tomatoes, chopped
Salt, to taste
1 French baguette, cut diagonally into 1-inch slices

1. Preheat the toaster oven to 400ºF (205ºC).
2. Process the mixture ingredients in a blender or food processor until smooth.
3. Spread the mixture on both sides of each bread slice, reassemble into a loaf, and wrap in aluminum foil.
4. Bake for 12 minutes, or until the bread is thoroughly heated. Peel back the aluminum foil to expose the top of the bread.
5. Bake again for 5 minutes, or until the top is lightly browned.

Honey Banana Bread

Prep time: 10 minutes | Cook time: 40 minutes | Serves 6

2 ripe bananas
1 egg
½ cup milk
2 tablespoons honey
2 tablespoons vegetable oil
¾ cup chopped trail mix
1 cup unbleached flour
1 teaspoon baking powder
Pinch of salt

1. Preheat the toaster oven to 400ºF (205ºC).
2. Process the bananas, egg, milk, honey, and oil in a blender or food processor until smooth. Pour into a mixing bowl.
3. Add the flour and trail mix, stirring to mix well. Add the baking powder and salt and stir just enough to blend. Pour the mixture into an oiled or nonstick regular-size 8½ × 4½ × 2¼-inch loaf pan.
4. Bake for 40 minutes, or until a knife inserted in the center comes out clean.

CHAPTER 8 PIZZA

Two Yeast Pizza Dough

Prep time: 5 minutes | Cook time: 20 minutes | Makes 2 9-inch pizza crusts

¼ cup tepid water
1 cup tepid skim milk
½ teaspoon sugar
1 (1¼-ounce / 35.4-g) envelope dry yeast
2 cups unbleached flour
1 tablespoon olive oil

1. Preheat the toaster oven to 400ºF (205ºC).
2. Combine the water, milk, and sugar in a bowl. Add the yeast and set aside for 3 to 5 minutes, or until the yeast is dissolved.
3. Stir in the flour gradually, adding just enough to form a ball of the dough.
4. Knead on a floured surface until the dough is satiny, and then put the dough in a bowl in a warm place with a damp towel over the top. In 1 hour or when the dough has doubled in bulk, punch it down and divide it in half. Flatten the dough and spread it out to the desired thickness on an oiled or nonstick 9¾-inch-diameter pie pan. Spread with your favorite pizza sauce and add any desired toppings.
5. Bake for 20 minutes, or until the topping ingredients are cooked and the cheese is melted.

Chicken and Tomato Cheese Pizza

Prep time: 10 minutes | Cook time: 25 minutes | Serves 4

1 (9-inch) ready-made pizza crust
1 (8-ounce / 227-g) can tomato sauce
1 tablespoon olive oil
1 cup skinless, boneless chicken breast, cooked and cubed
3 plum tomatoes, chopped
1 bell pepper, quartered, seeded, and chopped
2 garlic cloves, minced
½ teaspoon dried oregano
½ teaspoon dried basil
½ teaspoon red pepper flakes
1 cup shredded part-skim, low-moisture Mozzarella cheese

1. Preheat the toaster oven to 400ºF (205ºC).
2. Spread the pizza crust with the tomato sauce. Drizzle with the olive oil and sprinkle with the chicken, tomatoes, pepper, garlic, seasonings, and cheese. Place the pizza on the toaster oven rack.
3. Bake for 25 minutes, or until the topping is cooked and the crust is lightly browned.

Italian Mozzarella Vegetable Pizza

Prep time: 10 minutes | Cook time: 30 minutes | Serves 4

½ cup tomato sauce
2 tablespoons tomato paste
2 tablespoons olive oil
½ cup grated zucchini
½ cup grated onion
2 tablespoons grated bell pepper
1 teaspoon garlic powder
2 tablespoons chopped pitted black olives
1 teaspoon dried oregano
Salt, to taste
¼ cup Mozzarella cheese

1. Preheat the toaster oven to 375ºF (190ºC).
2. Cut the loaf of bread in half lengthwise, then in quarters crosswise. Remove some of the bread from the center to make a cavity for the pizza topping.
3. Combine all the topping ingredients and spoon equal portions into the cavities in the bread. Sprinkle with Mozzarella cheese. Place the bread quarters on the toaster oven rack.
4. Bake for 30 minutes, or until the cheese is melted and the crust is lightly browned.

Sun-Dried Tomato and Mushroom Pizza

Prep time: 10 minutes | Cook time: 32 minutes | Serves 4

1 cup chopped sun-dried tomatoes
2 tablespoons tomato paste
2 tablespoons olive oil
2 tablespoons chopped onion
2 garlic cloves, minced

1 teaspoon dried oregano
1 teaspoon dried basil
Salt and red pepper flakes, to taste
1 (9-inch) ready-made pizza crust
1 (5-ounce / 142-g) can mushrooms
¼ cup pitted and sliced black olives
½ cup shredded low-fat Mozzarella cheese

1. Combine the tomato mixture ingredients with ½ cup water in an 8½ × 8½ × 2-inch square baking (cake) pan.
2. Broil for 8 minutes, or until the tomatoes are softened. Remove from the oven and cool for 5 minutes.
3. Process the mixture in a blender or food processor until well blended. Spread on the pizza crust and layer with the mushrooms, olives, and cheese.
4. Bake at 400ºF (205ºC). for 25 minutes, or until the cheese is melted.

Oregano Turkey and Artichoke Pizza

Prep time: 10 minutes | Cook time: 30 minutes | Serves 1

1 (9-inch) ready-made pizza crust
1 teaspoon olive oil
2 tablespoons tomato paste
4 ounces (113 g) ground lean turkey breast
2 tablespoons sliced marinated artichokes
2 tablespoons pitted and chopped Kalamata olives
2 tablespoons crumbled Feta cheese
1 tablespoon chopped fresh basil leaves
1 tablespoon chopped fresh oregano leaves
2 tablespoons grated Parmesan cheese
¼ teaspoon red pepper flakes

1. Preheat the toaster oven to 375ºF (190ºC).
2. Brush the pizza crust with the olive oil and spread on the tomato paste. Add all the other ingredients. Place the pizza on the toaster oven rack.
3. Bake for 30 minutes, or until the topping is cooked and the crust is lightly browned.

Quick Pizza

Prep time: 5 minutes | Cook time: 3 minutes | Serves 1

2 tablespoons salsa
1 (6-inch) whole wheat pita bread
2 tablespoons shredded part-skim, low-moisture Mozzarella cheese

1. Spread the salsa on the pita bread and sprinkle with the cheese.
2. Bake once, or until the cheese is melted.

Herb Bell Pepper Cheese Pizza

Prep time: 15 minutes | Cook time: 25 minutes | Serves 4

1 (9-inch) ready-made pizza crust
1 tablespoon olive oil
1 (4-ounce / 113-g) can tomato paste
2 tablespoons shredded part-skim Mozzarella
2 tablespoons grated Parmesan cheese
2 tablespoons crumbled Feta cheese
½ bell pepper, chopped
1 tablespoon chopped fresh parsley
1 tablespoon chopped fresh oregano
1 tablespoon chopped fresh basil
½ teaspoon red pepper flakes
Salt and freshly ground black pepper, to taste
Pizza Mixture:
2 garlic cloves, minced
1 plum tomato, chopped

1. Preheat the toaster oven to 400ºF (205ºC).
2. Brush the pizza crust with olive oil and spread the tomato paste evenly to cover.
3. Combine the ingredients for the pizza mixture and spread evenly on top of the tomato paste layer. Sprinkle the cheeses over all and season to taste. Place the pizza on the toaster oven rack.
4. Bake for 25 minutes, or until the vegetables are cooked and the cheese is melted.

Super Cheesy Pesto Pizza

Prep time: 10 minutes | Cook time: 20 minutes | Serves 1

½ cup chopped fresh basil
1 tablespoon pine nuts (pignoli)
1 tablespoon olive oil
2 tablespoons shredded Parmesan cheese
1 garlic clove, minced
½ teaspoon dried oregano or 1 tablespoon chopped fresh oregano

1 plum tomato, chopped
Salt and pepper to taste
1 (9-inch) ready-made pizza crust
2 tablespoons shredded low-fat Mozzarella

1. Preheat the toaster oven to 375ºF (190ºC).
2. Combine the topping ingredients in a small bowl.
3. Process the mixture in a blender or food processor until smooth. Spread the mixture on the pizza crust, then sprinkle with the Mozzarella cheese. Place the pizza crust on the toaster oven rack.
4. Bake for 20 minutes, or until the cheese is melted and the crust is brown.

Spinach and Tomato Cheese Pizza

Prep time: 10 minutes | Cook time: 30 minutes | Serves 2

8 sheets phyllo dough, thawed and folded in half
4 tablespoons olive oil
4 tablespoons grated Parmesan cheese

Topping Mixture:

1 (10-ounce / 283-g) package frozen chopped spinach, thawed and well drained
1 plum tomato, finely chopped
¼ cup finely chopped onion
¼ cup shredded low-fat Mozzarella cheese
3 tablespoons crumbled Feta cheese or part-skim ricotta cheese
2 garlic cloves, minced
Salt and freshly ground black pepper, to taste

1. Preheat the toaster oven to 375ºF (190ºC).
2. Layer the sheets of phyllo dough in an oiled or nonstick 9¾-inch-diameter baking pan, lightly brushing the top of each sheet with olive oil and folding in the corner edges to fit the pan.
3. Combine the topping mixture ingredients in a bowl and adjust the seasonings to taste. Spread the mixture on top of the phyllo pastry layers and sprinkle with the Parmesan cheese.
4. Bake for 30 minutes, or until the cheese is melted and the topping is lightly browned. Remove carefully from the pan with a metal spatula.

CHAPTER 9 SOUP

Narragansett Clam Chowder with Parsley

Prep time: 10 minutes | Cook time:minutes | Serves 4

1 cup fat-free half-and-half
2 tablespoons unbleached flour
3½ cup chopped onion
1 cup peeled and diced potato
1 tablespoon vegetable oil
1 tablespoon chopped fresh parsley
1 (6-ounce / 170-g) can clams, drained and chopped
1 (15-ounce / 425-g) can fat-free low-sodium chicken broth
Salt and freshly ground black pepper, to taste

1. Whisk together the half-and-half and flour in a small bowl. Set aside.
2. Combine the onion, potato, and oil in an 8½ × 8½ × 2-inch square baking (cake) pan.
3. Broil 15 minutes, turning every 5 minutes with tongs, or until the potato is tender and the onion is cooked. Transfer to a 1-quart baking dish. Add the parsley, clams, broth, and half-and-half and flour mixture. Stir well and season to taste with salt and pepper.
4. Bake, uncovered, at 375ºF (190ºC). for 20 minutes, stirring after 10 minutes, or until the stock is reduced and thickened. Ladle into bowls and serve.

French Bread on Cheesy Onion Soup

Prep time: 10 minutes | Cook time: 46 minutes | Serves 4

1 cup finely chopped onions
1 teaspoon toasted sesame oil
1 tablespoon vegetable oil
2½ cup dry white wine
3 teaspoons soy sauce
½ teaspoon garlic powder
Freshly ground black pepper, to taste
4 French bread rounds, sliced 1 inch thick
4 tablespoons grated Parmesan cheese
1 tablespoon chopped fresh parsley

1. Place the onions, sesame oil, and vegetable oil in an 8½ × 8½ × 2-inch square baking (cake) pan.
2. Broil for 10 minutes, stirring every 3 minutes until the onions are tender. Remove from the oven and transfer to a 1-quart 8½ × 8½ × 4-inch ovenproof baking dish. Add 2 cups water, the wine, and the soy sauce. Add the garlic powder and pepper and adjust the seasonings.
3. Bake, covered, at 400ºF (205ºC). for 30 minutes. Remove from the oven, uncover, and add the 4 bread rounds, letting them float on top of the soup. Sprinkle each with 1 tablespoon Parmesan cheese.
4. Broil, uncovered, for 6 minutes, or until the cheese is lightly browned. With tongs, transfer the bread rounds to 4 individual soup bowls. Ladle the soup on top of the bread rounds. Garnish with the parsley and serve immediately.

Gazpacho

Prep time: 15 minutes | Cook time: 35 minutes | Serves 4

1 bell pepper, thinly sliced
½ cup chopped celery
½ cup frozen or canned corn
1 medium onion, thinly sliced
1 small yellow squash, cut into 1-inch slices
1 small zucchini, cut into 1-inch slices
3 garlic cloves, chopped
½ teaspoon ground cumin
2 tablespoons olive oil
Salt and freshly ground black pepper, to taste
1 quart tomato juice
1 tablespoon lemon juice
3 tablespoons chopped fresh cilantro

1. Preheat the toaster oven to 400ºF (205ºC).
2. Combine the vegetables and seasonings in an oiled or nonstick 8½ × 8½ × 2-inch square baking (cake) pan, mixing well.
3. Bake, covered, for 25 minutes, or until the onions and celery are tender. Remove from the oven, uncover, and turn the vegetable pieces with tongs.

4. Broil for 10 minutes, or until the vegetables are lightly browned. Remove from the oven and cool. Transfer to a large nonaluminum container and add the tomato juice, lemon juice, and cilantro. Adjust the seasonings.

5. Chill, covered, for several hours, preferably a day or two to enrich the flavor of the stock.

Pea and Turkey Bacon Soup

Prep time: 10 minutes | Cook time: 55 minutes | Serves 6

1 cup dried split peas, ground in a blender to a powder like consistency
3 strips lean turkey bacon, uncooked and chopped
¼ cup grated carrots
¼ cup grated celery
2 tablespoons grated onion
½ teaspoon garlic powder
Salt and freshly ground black pepper, to taste
2 tablespoons chopped fresh chives, for garnish

1. Preheat the toaster oven to 400ºF (205ºC).
2. Combine all the ingredients in a 1-quart 8½ × 8½ × 4-inch ovenproof baking dish, mixing well. Adjust the seasonings.
3. Bake, covered, for 35 minutes. Remove from the oven and stir.
4. Bake, covered, for another 20 minutes, or until the soup is thickened. Ladle the soup into individual soup bowls and garnish each with chopped fresh chives.

Connecticut Chowder

Prep time: 15 minutes | Cook time: 1 hour | Serves 4

Soup:

½ cup peeled and shredded potato
½ cup shredded carrot
½ cup shredded celery
2 plum tomatoes, chopped
1 small zucchini, shredded
2 bay leaves
¼ teaspoon sage
1 teaspoon garlic powder
Salt and butcher's pepper, to taste

Chowder Base:

2 tablespoons reduced-fat cream cheese, at room temperature
½ cup fat-free half-and-half
2 tablespoons unbleached flour
2 tablespoons chopped fresh parsley

1. Preheat the toaster oven to 375ºF (190ºC).
2. Combine the soup ingredients in a 1-quart 8½ × 8½ × 4-inch ovenproof baking dish, mixing well. Adjust the seasonings to taste.
3. Bake, covered, for 40 minutes, or until the vegetables are tender.
4. Whisk the chowder mixture ingredients together until smooth. Add the mixture to the cooked soup ingredients and stir well to blend.
5. Bake, uncovered for 20 minutes, or until the stock is thickened. Ladle the soup into individual soup bowls and garnish with the parsley.

Crab and Vegetable Chowder

Prep time: 15 minutes | Cook time: 40 minutes | Serves 4

1 (6-ounce / 170-g) can lump crab meat, drained and chopped
1 cup skim milk or low-fat soy milk
1 cup fat-free half-and-half
2 tablespoons unbleached flour
¼ cup chopped onion
½ cup peeled and diced potato
1 carrot, peeled and chopped
1 celery stalk, chopped
2 garlic cloves, minced
2 tablespoons chopped fresh parsley
½ teaspoon ground cumin
1 teaspoon paprika
Salt and butcher's pepper, to taste

1. Preheat the toaster oven to 400ºF (205ºC).
2. Whisk together the milk, half-and-half, and flour in a bowl. Transfer the mixture to a 1-quart 8½ × 8½ × 4-inch ovenproof baking dish. Add all the other ingredients, mixing well. Adjust the seasonings to taste.
3. Bake, covered, for 40 minutes, or until the vegetables are tender.

Oregano Green Bean Soup

Prep time: 10 minutes | Cook time: 47 minutes | Serves 4

2 tablespoons unbleached flour
1 tablespoon margarine
3 cups water or low-sodium vegetable stock
1 cup fresh string beans, trimmed and cut into 1-inch pieces
½ teaspoon dried oregano
½ teaspoon ground cumin
Salt and freshly ground black pepper, to taste

1. Combine the roux mixture in an 8½ × 8½ × 2-inch baking (cake) pan.
2. Broil for 5 minutes, or until the margarine is melted. Remove from the oven and stir, then broil again for 2 minutes, or until the mixture is brown but not burned. Remove from the oven and stir to mix well. Set aside.
3. Combine the water or broth, string beans, and seasonings in a 1-quart 8½ × 8½ × 4-inch ovenproof baking dish. Stir in the roux mixture, blending well. Adjust the seasonings to taste.
4. Bake, covered, at 375ºF (190ºC). for 40 minutes, or until the string beans are tender.

Lentil, Carrot and Mushroom Soup

Prep time: 10 minutes | Cook time: 40 minutes | Serves 4

½ cup lentils
½ cup dry white wine
1 small onion, chopped
3 carrots, peeled and finely chopped
½ cup fresh mushrooms, cleaned and sliced
3 garlic cloves, minced
1 tablespoon chopped fresh parsley
1 tablespoon Worcestershire sauce
Salt and freshly ground black pepper, to taste

1. Preheat the toaster oven to 375ºF (190ºC).
2. Combine all the ingredients with 2 cups water in a 1-quart 8½ × 8½ × 4-inch ovenproof baking dish. Adjust the seasonings.
3. Bake for 40 minutes, or until the lentils, carrots, and onions are tender. Ladle into individual soup bowls and serve.

Chicken and Vegetable Noodle Soup

Prep time: 10 minutes | Cook time: 45 minutes | Serves 4

1 cup egg noodles, uncooked
1 skinless, boneless chicken breast filet, cut into 1-inch pieces
1 carrot, peeled and chopped
1 celery stalk, chopped
1 plum tomato, chopped
1 small onion, peeled and chopped
1 tablespoon chopped fresh parsley
1 teaspoon dried basil
Salt and freshly ground black pepper, to taste

1. Preheat the toaster oven to 400ºF (205ºC).
2. Combine all the ingredients with 3 cups water in a 1-quart 8½ × 8½ × 4-inch ovenproof baking dish.
3. Bake, covered, for 45 minutes, or until the vegetables and chicken are tender.

Creamy Roasted Peppers Soup

Prep time: 10 minutes | Cook time: 35 minutes | Serves 4

1 (5-ounce / 142-g) jar roasted peppers, drained
½ cup fresh basil leaves
1 cup fat-free half-and-half
1 cup skim milk
2 tablespoons reduced-fat cream cheese
1 teaspoon garlic powder
1 teaspoon paprika
Salt and freshly ground black pepper, to taste
2 tablespoons chopped fresh basil leaves (garnish for cold soup)
2 tablespoons grated Parmesan cheese (topping for hot soup)

1. Preheat the toaster oven to 400ºF (205ºC).
2. Process all the ingredients in a blender or food processor until smooth. Transfer the mixture to a 1-quart 8½ × 8½ × 4-inch ovenproof baking dish.

3. Bake, covered, for 35 minutes. Ladle into individual soup bowls and serve.

Tomato Bisque with Basil

Prep time: 10 minutes | Cook time: 25 minutes | Serves 4

1 (8-ounce / 227-g) can tomato sauce
1 (7-ounce / 198-g) jar diced pimientos, drained
1 tablespoon finely chopped onion
2 cups low-fat buttermilk
1 cup fat-free half-and-half
1 tablespoon low-fat cream cheese
1 teaspoon garlic powder
½ teaspoon paprika
½ teaspoon ground bay leaf
1 teaspoon hot sauce (optional)
Salt and white pepper to taste
2 tablespoons minced fresh basil leaves

1. Preheat the toaster oven to 350ºF (180ºC).
2. Process all the ingredients except the basil in a blender or food processor until smooth. Pour into a 1-quart 8½ × 8½ × 4-inch ovenproof baking dish. Adjust the seasonings to taste.
3. Bake, covered, for 25 minutes. Ladle into small soup bowls and garnish each with fresh basil leaves before serving.

CHAPTER 10 GRAINS

Gardener's Vegetable Rice

Prep time: 10 minutes | Cook time: 30 minutes | Serves 4

½ cup rice
2 tablespoons finely chopped scallions
2 small zucchini, finely chopped
1 bell pepper, finely chopped
1 small tomato, finely chopped
¼ cup frozen peas
¼ cup frozen corn
1 teaspoon ground cumin
½ teaspoon dried oregano
Salt and freshly ground black pepper, to taste

1. Preheat the toaster oven to 400ºF (205ºC).
2. Combine all the ingredients with ¼ cups water in a 1-quart 8½ × 8½ × 4-inch ovenproof baking dish, stirring well to blend. Adjust the seasonings to taste. Cover with aluminum foil.
3. Bake, covered, for 30 minutes, or until the rice and vegetables are almost cooked. Remove from the oven, uncover, and let stand for 10 minutes to complete the cooking. Fluff once more and adjust the seasonings before serving.

Moroccan Vegetable Couscous

Prep time: 10 minutes | Cook time: 12 minutes | Serves 4

1 cup couscous
2 tablespoons finely chopped scallion
2 tablespoons finely chopped bell pepper
1 plum tomato, finely chopped
2 tablespoons chopped pitted black olives
1 tablespoon olive oil
¼ teaspoon ground cumin
¼ teaspoon ground cinnamon
¼ teaspoon turmeric
Pinch of cayenne
Salt and freshly ground black pepper, to taste

1. Preheat the toaster oven to 400ºF (205ºC).
2. Combine all the ingredients with ¼ cups water in a 1-quart 8½ × 8½ × 4-inch ovenproof baking dish. Adjust the seasonings to taste. Cover with aluminum foil.
3. Bake, covered, for 12 minutes. Remove from the heat and fluff with a fork. Cover again and let stand for 10 minutes. Fluff once more before serving.

Couscous with Chickpeas and Green Peas

Prep time: 10 minutes | Cook time: 10 minutes | Serves 4

1 (10-ounce / 283-g) package couscous
2 tablespoons olive oil
2 tablespoons canned chickpeas
2 tablespoons canned or frozen green peas
1 tablespoon chopped fresh parsley
3 scallions, chopped
Salt and pepper, to taste

1. Preheat the toaster oven to 400ºF (205ºC).
2. Mix together all the ingredients with 2 cups water in a 1-quart 8½ × 8½ × 4-inch ovenproof baking dish. Adjust the seasonings to taste. Cover with aluminum foil.
3. Bake, covered, for 10 minutes, or until the couscous and vegetables are tender. Adjust the seasonings to taste and fluff with a fork before serving.

Lush Veggies Salad

Prep time: 10 minutes | Cook time: 35 minutes | Serves

¼ cup lentils
1 tablespoon olive oil

For the Salad:

1 celery stalk, trimmed and chopped
1 plum tomato, chopped
1 cucumber, peeled, seeded, and chopped
1½ cups spinach leaves, pulled into small pieces
1 tablespoon balsamic vinegar
1 tablespoon olive oil
½ teaspoon dried oregano
1 tablespoon chopped scallions
2 tablespoons sliced pitted black olives
1 teaspoon minced roasted garlic

1. Preheat the toaster oven to 400ºF (205ºC).

2. Combine the lentils, ¼ cups water, and olive oil in a 1-quart 8½ × 8½ × 4-inch ovenproof baking dish. Cover with aluminum foil.
3. Bake, covered, for 35 minutes, or until the lentils are tender. When cool, combine with all the salad ingredients in a serving bowl and toss well. Adjust the seasonings, chill, and serve.

Sesame Barley

Prep time: 5 minutes | Cook time: 50 minutes | Serves 2

$^{1}/_{3}$ cup barley, toasted
1 tablespoon sesame oil
1 tablespoon sesame seeds
¼ teaspoon ground cumin
¼ teaspoon turmeric
½ teaspoon garlic powder
Salt and freshly ground black pepper, to taste

1. Combine the barley and 1½ cups water in a 1-quart 8½ × 8½ × 4-inch ovenproof baking dish. Cover with aluminum foil.
2. Bake, covered, for 50 minutes, or until almost cooked, testing the grains after 30 minutes for softness.
3. Add the oil and seasonings and fluff with a fork to combine. Cover and let the barley sit for 10 minutes to finish cooking and absorb the flavors of the seasonings. Fluff once more before serving.

Fat-Free Salad Couscous

Prep time: 10 minutes | Cook time: 10 minutes | Serves 4

1 (10-ounce / 283-g) package precooked couscous
2 tablespoons olive oil
Salt and freshly ground black pepper, to taste
¼ cup chopped fresh tomatoes
2 tablespoons chopped fresh basil leaves
1 tablespoon sliced almonds
½ bell pepper, chopped
3 scallions, chopped
2 tablespoons lemon juice

1. Preheat the toaster oven to 400ºF (205ºC).
2. Mix together the couscous, 2 cups water, and olive oil in a 1-quart 8½ × 8½ × 4-inch ovenproof baking dish. Add salt and pepper to taste. Cover with aluminum foil.
3. Bake, covered, for 10 minutes, or until the couscous is cooked. Remove from the oven, fluff with a fork and, when cool, add the tomatoes, basil leaves, almonds, pepper, scallions, and lemon juice. Adjust the seasonings to taste. Chill before serving.

Oven-Baked Spanish Rice

Prep time: 10 minutes | Cook time: 45 minutes | Serves 4

¾ cup rice
2 tablespoons dry white wine
3 tablespoons olive oil
1 (15-ounce / 425-g) can whole tomatoes
¼ cup thinly sliced onions
3 tablespoons chopped fresh cilantro
4½ cup chopped bell pepper
5 bay leaves
Salt and a pinch of red pepper flakes, to taste

1. Preheat the toaster oven to 375ºF (190ºC).
2. Combine all the ingredients with 1 cup water in a 1-quart 8½ × 8½ × 4-inch ovenproof baking dish and adjust the seasonings. Cover with aluminum foil.
3. Bake, covered, for 45 minutes, or until the rice is cooked, removing the cover after 30 minutes.

Simple Oven-Baked Rice

Prep time: 5 minutes | Cook time: 30 minutes | Serves 2

¼ cup regular rice (not parboiled or precooked)
1 tablespoon olive oil
1 teaspoon dried parsley
1 teaspoon garlic powder
Salt and freshly ground black pepper, to taste

1. Preheat the toaster oven to 400ºF (205ºC).
2. Combine ¼ cups water and the rice in a 1-quart 8½ × 8½ × 4-inch ovenproof baking dish. Stir well to blend. Cover with aluminum foil.
3. Bake, covered, for 30 minutes, or until the rice is almost cooked. Add the seasonings, fluff with a fork to combine the seasonings well, then let the rice sit, covered, for 10 minutes. Fluff once more before serving.

Buttermilk Garlicky Lentils

Prep time: 10 minutes | Cook time: 35 minutes | Serves 2

¼ cup lentils
1 tablespoon mashed roasted garlic
1 rosemary sprig
1 bay leaf
Salt and freshly ground black pepper, to taste
2 tablespoons low-fat buttermilk
2 tablespoons tomato sauce

1. Preheat the toaster oven to 400ºF (205ºC).
2. Combine the lentils, 1¼ cups water, garlic, rosemary sprig, and bay leaf in a 1-quart 8½ × 8½ × 4-inch ovenproof baking dish, stirring to blend well. Add the salt and pepper to taste. Cover with aluminum foil.
3. Bake, covered, for 35 minutes, or until the lentils are tender. Remove the rosemary sprig and bay leaf and stir in the buttermilk and tomato sauce. Serve immediately.

Sweet Kasha Loaf

Prep time: 10 minutes | Cook time: 30 minutes | Serves 4

1 cup whole grain kasha
2 cups tomato sauce
3 tablespoons minced onion or scallions
1 tablespoon minced garlic
1 cup multigrain bread crumbs
1 egg
1 teaspoon paprika
1 teaspoon chili powder
1 teaspoon sesame oil

1. Preheat the toaster oven to 400ºF (205ºC).
2. Combine all the ingredients in a bowl and transfer to an oiled or nonstick regular-size 4½ × 8½ × 2/4-inch loaf pan.
3. Bake, uncovered, for 30 minutes, or until lightly browned.

Kasha Burger

Prep time: 10 minutes | Cook time: 30 minutes | Serves 4

1 cup kasha
2 tablespoons minced onion or scallions
1 tablespoon minced garlic
½ cup multigrain bread crumbs
1 egg
¼ teaspoon paprika
½ teaspoon chili powder
¼ teaspoon sesame oil
1 tablespoon vegetable oil
Salt and freshly ground black pepper, to taste

1. Preheat the toaster oven to 400ºF (205ºC).
2. Combine 2 cups water and the kasha in a 1-quart 8½ × 8½ × 4-inch ovenproof baking dish.
3. Bake, uncovered, for 30 minutes, or until the grains are cooked. Remove from the oven and add all the other ingredients, stirring to mix well. When the mixture is cooled, shape into 4 to 6 patties and place on a rack with a broiling pan underneath.
4. Broil for 20 minutes, turn with a spatula, then broil for another 10 minutes, or until browned.

Parmesan Turkey Bacon Grits

Prep time: 10 minutes | Cook time: 30 minutes | Serves 4

4 strips lean uncooked turkey bacon, cut in half
1 cup grits
2 cups skim or low-fat soy milk
1 egg
½ cup shredded Parmesan cheese
1 tablespoon chopped fresh parsley
½ teaspoon garlic powder
Salt and butcher's pepper, to taste

1. Preheat the toaster oven to 350ºF (180ºC).
2. Layer an 8½ × 8½ × 2-inch square baking (cake) pan with the bacon strips.
3. Combine the remaining ingredients in a medium bowl and pour the mixture over the strips.
4. Bake, uncovered, for 30 minutes, or until the grits are cooked. Cut into squares with a spatula and serve.

APPENDIX : RECIPES INDEX

Milton Keynes UK
Ingram Content Group UK Ltd.
UKHW051909231023
431198UK00002B/17

9 781802 443936